Addressing Violence in Pediatric Practice

Editors

JOEL A. FEIN
MEGAN H. BAIR-MERRITT

PEDIATRIC CLINICS
OF NORTH AMERICA

www.pediatric.theclinics.com

Consulting Editor
TINA L. CHENG

December 2023 • Volume 70 • Number 6

ELSEVIER

1600 John F. Kennedy Boulevard • Suite 1800 • Philadelphia, Pennsylvania, 19103-2899

http://www.theclinics.com

THE PEDIATRIC CLINICS OF NORTH AMERICA Volume 70, Number 6
December 2023 ISSN 0031-3955, ISBN-13: 978-0-443-18304-1

Editor: Kerry Holland
Developmental Editor: Saswoti Nath

The Pediatric Clinics of North America (ISSN 0031-3955) is published bimonthly by Elsevier Inc., 360 Park Avenue South, New York, NY 10010-1710. Months of issue are February, April, June, August, October, and December. Periodicals postage paid at New York, NY and additional mailing offices. Subscription prices are $279.00 per year (US individuals), $827.00 per year (US institutions), $351.00 per year (Canadian individuals), $1100.00 per year (Canadian institutions), $419.00 per year (international individuals), $1100.00 per year (international institutions), $100.00 per year (US students and residents), $100.00 per year (Canadian students and residents), and $165.00 per year (international residents and students). To receive students/resident rare, orders must be accompanied by name of affiliated institution, date of term, and the signature of program/residency coordinator on institution letterhead. Orders will be billed at individual rate until proof of status is received. Foreign air speed delivery is included in all *Clinics* subscription prices. All prices are subject to change without notice. **POSTMASTER:** Send address changes to *The Pediatric Clinics of North America*, Elsevier Health Sciences Division, Subscription Customer Service, 3251 Riverport Lane, Maryland Heights, MO 63043. **Customer Service: 1-800-654-2452 (US and Canada). From outside of the US and Canada: 1-314-447-8871. Fax: 1-314-447-8029. For print support, E-mail: JournalsCustomerService-usa@elsevier. com. For online support, E-mail: JournalsOnlineSupport-usa@elsevier.com.**

Reprints. For copies of 100 or more, of articles in this publication, please contact the Commercial Reprints Department, Elsevier Inc., 360 Park Avenue South, New York, NY 10010-1710. Tel.: 212-633-3874; Fax: 212-633-3820; E-mail: reprints@elsevier.com.

The Pediatric Clinics of North America is also published in Spanish by McGraw-Hill Inter-americana Editores S.A., Mexico City, Mexico; in Portuguese by Riechmann and Affonso Editores, Rua Comandante Coelho 1085, CEP 21250, Rio de Janeiro, Brazil; and in Greek by Althayia SA, Athens, Greece.

The Pediatric Clinics of North America is covered in *MEDLINE/PubMed (Index Medicus), Excerpta Medica, Current Contents, Current Contents/Clinical Medicine, Science Citation Index, ASCA, ISI/BIOMED,* and *BIOSIS*.

PROGRAM OBJECTIVE

The goal of the *Pediatric Clinics of North America* is to keep practicing physicians and residents up to date with current clinical practice in pediatrics by providing timely articles reviewing the state-of-the-art in patient care.

TARGET AUDIENCE

All practicing pediatricians, physicians, and healthcare professionals who provide patient care to pediatric patients.

LEARNING OBJECTIVES

Upon completion of this activity, participants will be able to:

1. Review how pediatric healthcare providers create healing spaces to support survivors of intimate partner violence (IPV) and their children.
2. Discuss preventative measures associated with unintentional firearm injuries.
3. Recognize the long-term physical and mental health consequences of bullying, especially for vulnerable youth.

ACCREDITATIONS

Physician Credit

The Elsevier Office of Continuing Medical Education (EOCME) is accredited by the Accreditation Council for Continuing Medical Education (ACCME) to provide continuing medical education for physicians.

The EOCME designates this journal-based activity for a maximum of 13 *AMA PRA Category 1 Credit*(s)™. Physicians should claim only the credit commensurate with the extent of their participation in the activity.

All other healthcare professionals requesting continuing education credit for this journal-based activity will be issued a certificate of participation.

ABP Maintenance of Certification Credit

Successful completion of this CME activity, which includes participation in the activity and individual assessment of and feedback to the learner, enables the learner to earn up to 13 MOC points in the American Board of Pediatrics' (ABP) Maintenance of Certification (MOC) program. It is the CME activity provider's responsibility to submit learner completion information to ACCME for the purpose of granting ABP MOC credit.

DISCLOSURE OF CONFLICTS OF INTEREST

The EOCME assesses conflict of interest with its instructors, faculty, planners, and other individuals who are in a position to control the content of CME activities. All relevant conflicts of interest that are identified are thoroughly vetted by EOCME for fair balance, scientific objectivity, and patient care recommendations. EOCME is committed to providing its learners with CME activities that promote improvements or quality in healthcare and not a specific proprietary business or a commercial interest.

The planning committee, staff, authors, and editors listed below have identified no financial relationships or relationships to products or devices they or their spouse/life partner have with commercial interest related to the content of this CME activity:

Michael Arenson, MD, MS, MA; Megan Bair-Merritt, MD, MSCE; Steven Berkowitz, MD; Rhonda C. Boyd, PhD; Brad J. Bushman, PhD; Eduard Coupet, MD, MS; Alison J. Culyba, MD, PHD, MPH; Molly Davis, PhD; James Dodington, MD; Katie A. Donnelly, MD, MPH; Jeremy Esposito, MD, MSEd; Joel Fein, MD, MPH; Daniel J. Flannery, PhD; Eric W. Fleegler, MD, MPH; Heather Forkey, MD; Kelsey A.B. Gastineau, MD; Monika K. Goyal, MD, MSCE; Yuan He, MD, MPH, MSHP; Jennifer Hoffmann, MD, MS; Lenore Jarvis, MD, MEd; Samaa Kemal, MD, MPH; Caroline J. Kistin, MD, MSc; Lois K. Lee, MD, MPH; Michelle Littlejohn; Rajkumar Mayakrishnan, BSc, MBA; Amber R. McDonald, PhD, LCSW; Sandra McKay, MD; Ashlee Murray, MD, MPH; Laurel Niep, LCSW; Ivette Noriega, PhD; Adaobi Nwabuo, MBBS, MPH; Abdullah H. Pratt, MD; Maya I. Ragavan, MD, MPH, MS; Uma Raman, MD; Kimberly A. Randell, MD, MSc; Michael Rich, MD, MPH; Dan Romer, PhD; Seth Scholer, MD; Ashley Sward, PsyD, IMH-E®; Destiny G. Tolliver, MD, MHS; Jodi Zik, MD

The planning committee, staff, authors, and editors listed below have identified financial relationships or relationships to products or devices they or their spouse/life partner have with commercial interest related to the content of this CME activity:

UNAPPROVED/OFF-LABEL USE DISCLOSURE

The EOCME requires CME faculty to disclose to the participants:

1. When products or procedures being discussed are off-label, unlabelled, experimental, and/or investigational (not US Food and Drug Administration [FDA] approved); and
2. Any limitations on the information presented, such as data that are preliminary or that represent ongoing research, interim analyses, and/or unsupported opinions. Faculty may discuss information about pharmaceutical agents that is outside of FDA-approved labelling. This information is intended solely for CME and is not intended to promote off-label use of these medications. If you have any questions, contact the medical affairs department of the manufacturer for the most recent prescribing information.

TO ENROLL

To enroll in the *Pediatric Clinics of North America* Continuing Medical Education program, call customer service at 1-800-654-2452 or sign up online at http://www.theclinics.com/home/cme. The CME program is available to subscribers for an additional annual fee of USD 214.00.

METHOD OF PARTICIPATION

In order to claim credit, participants must complete the following:

1. Complete enrolment as indicated above.
2. Read the activity.
3. Complete the CME Test and Evaluation. Participants must achieve a score of 70% on the test. All CME Tests and Evaluations must be completed online.

In order to claim MOC points, participants must complete the following:

1. Complete steps listed above for claiming CME credit
2. Provide your specialty board ID#, birth date (MM/DD), and attestation.
3. Online MOC submission is only available for the American Board of pediatrics' (ABP) Maintenance of Certification (MOC) program

CME INQUIRIES/SPECIAL NEEDS

For all CME inquiries or special needs, please contact elsevierCME@elsevier.com.

Contributors

CONSULTING EDITOR

TINA L. CHENG, MD, MPH
BK Rachford Professor and Chair of Pediatrics, University of Cincinnati, Director, Cincinnati Children's Research Foundation, Chief Medical Officer, Cincinnati Children's Hospital Medical Center, Cincinnati, Ohio

EDITORS

JOEL A. FEIN, MD, MPH
Professor of Pediatrics, Perelman School of Medicine, University of Pennsylvania, Attending Physician in Emergency Medicine and Co-Director, Center for Violence Prevention, Division of Emergency Medicine, Children's Hospital of Philadelphia, Philadelphia, Pennsylvania

MEGAN H. BAIR-MERRITT, MD, MSCE
Chief Scientific Officer and Vice President, Professor of Pediatrics, Boston Medical Center, Boston University Chobanian & Avedesian School of Medicine, Boston, Massachusetts

AUTHORS

MICHAEL ARENSON, MD, MS, MA
UMass Memorial Children's Medical Center, UMass Chan Medical School Research Fellow, Center for Child Health Equity, Worcester, Massachusetts

STEVEN BERKOWITZ, MD
Professor, Department of Psychiatry and Pediatrics, University of Colorado School of Medicine, Anschutz Medical Campus, Aurora, Colorado

RHONDA C. BOYD, PhD
Associate Professor, Department of Psychiatry, Perelman School of Medicine, University of Pennsylvania, Departments of Child and Adolescent Psychiatry and Behavioral Sciences and PolicyLab, Children's Hospital of Philadelphia, Philadelphia, Pennsylvania

BRAD J. BUSHMAN, PhD
Margaret Hall and Robert Randal Rinehart Chair of Mass Communication Professor, School of Communication, The Ohio State University, Columbus, Ohio

EDOUARD COUPET II, MD, MS
Assistant Professor of Emergency Medicine, Yale School of Medicine, Core Faculty, Addiction Medicine, New Haven, Connecticut

ALISON J. CULYBA, MD, PhD, MPH
Assistant Professor of Pediatrics, Division of Adolescent and Young Adult Medicine, UPMC Children's Hospital of Pittsburgh, University of Pittsburgh School of Medicine, Pittsburgh, Pennsylvania

MOLLY DAVIS, PhD
Assistant Professor, Department of Psychiatry, Perelman School of Medicine, Departments of Child and Adolescent Psychiatry and Behavioral Sciences and PolicyLab, Children's Hospital of Philadelphia, Penn Implementation Science Center at the Leonard Davis Institute of Health Economics (PISCE@LDI), University of Pennsylvania, Philadelphia, Pennsylvania

JAMES DODINGTON, MD
Associate Professor of Pediatrics and Emergency Medicine, Yale School of Medicine, Medical Director, Yale New Haven Center for Injury and Violence Prevention, New Haven, Connecticut

KATIE A. DONNELLY, MD, MPH
Associate Professor of Pediatrics and Emergency Medicine, Children's National Hospital, The George Washington University, Washington, DC

JEREMY ESPOSITO, MD, MSEd
Assistant Professor of Clinical Pediatrics, Division of Pediatric Emergency Medicine, Children's Hospital of Philadelphia, Departments of Pediatrics and Psychiatry, Perelman School of Medicine, University of Pennsylvania, Philadelphia, Pennsylvania

DANIEL J. FLANNERY, PhD
Dr. Semi J. and Ruth Begun Professor and Director, Begun Center for Violence Prevention, Research and Education, Jack, Joseph and Morton Mandel School of Applied Social Sciences, Professor of Pediatrics and Psychiatry, Case Western Reserve University, Cleveland, Ohio

ERIC W. FLEEGLER, MD, MPH
Associate Professor of Pediatrics and Emergency Medicine, Division of Emergency Medicine, Boston Children's Hospital, Harvard Medical School, Boston, Massachusetts

HEATHER FORKEY, MD
Professor, UMass Memorial Children's Medical Center, Center for Child Health Equity, Foster Children Evaluation Service (FaCES), Department of Pediatrics, University of Massachusetts Chan Medical School, Worcester, Massachusetts

KELSEY A.B. GASTINEAU, MD, MPH
Assistant Professor, Department of Pediatrics, Monroe Carell Jr Children's Hospital at Vanderbilt, Vanderbilt University Medical Center, Nashville, Tennessee

MONIKA K. GOYAL, MD, MSCE
Associate Professor of Pediatrics and Emergency Medicine, Children's National Hospital, The George Washington University, Washington, DC

YUAN HE, MD, MPH, MSHP
Division of General Pediatrics, Children's Hospital of Philadelphia, Department of Pediatrics, Perelman School of Medicine, University of Pennsylvania, Philadelphia, Pennsylvania

JENNIFER HOFFMANN, MD, MS
Assistant Professor, Division of Emergency Medicine, Ann & Robert H. Lurie Children's Hospital of Chicago, Department of Pediatrics, Northwestern University Feinberg School of Medicine, Chicago, Illinois

LENORE JARVIS, MD, MEd
Assistant Professor of Pediatrics, Children's National Hospital, The George Washington University School of Medicine and Health Sciences, Washington, DC

SAMAA KEMAL, MD, MPH
Fellow, Division of Emergency Medicine, Ann & Robert H. Lurie Children's Hospital of Chicago, Department of Pediatrics, Northwestern University Feinberg School of Medicine, Chicago, Illinois

CAROLINE J. KISTIN, MD, MSc
Associate Professor, Division of Health Services, Policy, and Practice, Hassenfeld Child Health and Innovation Institute, Brown University School of Public Health, Providence, Rhode Island

LOIS K. LEE, MD, MPH
Associate Professor of Pediatrics and Emergency Medicine, Division of Emergency Medicine, Boston Children's Hospital, Harvard Medical School, Boston, Massachusetts

AMBER R. MCDONALD, PhD, LCSW
Assistant Professor, Department of Psychiatry, University of Colorado School of Medicine, Anschutz Medical Campus, Aurora, Colorado

SANDRA MCKAY, MD
Associate Professor, Department of Pediatrics, McGovern Medical School, The University of Texas Health Science Center at Houston, Houston, Texas

ASHLEE MURRAY, MD, MPH
Division of Pediatric Emergency Medicine, Children's Hospital of Pennsylvania, Philadelphia, Pennsylvania

LAUREL NIEP, LCSW
Instructor, Department of Psychiatry, University of Colorado School of Medicine, Anschutz Medical Campus, Aurora, Colorado

IVETTE NORIEGA, PhD
Senior Research Associate, Begun Center for Violence Prevention, Research and Education, Jack, Joseph and Morton Mandel School of Applied Social Sciences, Case Western Reserve University, Cleveland, Ohio

ADAOBI NWABUO, MBBS, MPH
Department of Psychiatry and Behavioral Sciences, University of California Davis Health, Sacramento, California

ABDULLAH H. PRATT, MD
Assistant Professor of Emergency Medicine, Section of Emergency Medicine, The University of Chicago Medical Center, Chicago, Illinois

MAYA I. RAGAVAN, MD, MPH, MS
Assistant Professor, Division of General Academic Pediatrics, University of Pittsburgh, UPMC Children's Hospital of Pittsburgh, Pittsburgh, Pennsylvania

UMA RAMAN, MD
Clinical Fellow, Pediatric Critical Care, Yale New Haven Hospital, Yale School of Medicine, New Haven, Connecticut

KIMBERLY A. RANDELL, MD, MSc
Professor of Pediatrics, Children's Mercy Kansas City, University of Missouri-Kansas City School of Medicine, Kansas City, Missouri; University of Kansas School of Medicine, Kansas City, Kansas

MICHAEL RICH, MD, MPH
Associate Professor, Harvard Medical School, Digital Wellness Lab, Boston Children's Hospital, Boston, Massachusetts

DAN ROMER, PhD
Research Director, Annenberg Public Policy Center, University of Pennsylvania, Philadelphia, Pennsylvania

SETH J. SCHOLER, MD
Professor, Department of Pediatrics, Vanderbilt University Medical Center, Nashville, Tennessee

ASHLEY SWARD, PsyD, IMH-E
Assistant Professor, Department of Psychiatry, University of Colorado School of Medicine, Anschutz Medical Campus, Aurora, Colorado

DESTINY G. TOLLIVER, MD, MHS
Assistant Professor, Department of Pediatrics, Boston Medical Center, Boston University Chobanian & Avedisian School of Medicine, Boston, Massachusetts

JODI ZIK, MD
Senior Instructor, Department of Psychiatry and Pediatrics, University of Colorado School of Medicine, Anschutz Medical Campus, Aurora, Colorado

Contents

> Exposure to violence remains a significant issue for children in the United States. The COVID-19 pandemic exacerbated many of these exposures. Violence unequally impacts children of color and lesbian, gay, bisexual, transgender, and questioning youth. Pediatricians can and must continue to advocate and intervene to decrease pediatric violence exposure and its effects.

> Intimate partner violence (IPV) is a pervasive public health epidemic that influences child health and thriving. In this article, we discuss how pediatric healthcare providers and systems can create healing-centered spaces to support IPV survivors and their children. We review the use of universal education and resource provision to share information about IPV during all clinical encounters as a healing-centered alternative to screening. We also review how to support survivors who may share experiences of IPV, focused on validation, affirmation, and connection to resources. Clinicians are provided key action items to implement in their clinical settings.

> Adolescent relationship abuse (ARA) is highly prevalent across all sociodemographic groups with negative outcomes in multiple domains of health. Using a healing-centered engagement approach, health care providers can support healthy adolescent relationships and connect ARA survivors to resources and supports to ensure health and well-being. Essential components of health care support for adolescents experiencing ARA include validation of disclosure, assessing safety, a warm hand-off to advocacy resources, addressing immediate and long-term health needs, and connection to a trusted adult. Informing adolescents about limits of confidentiality and use of shared decision-making after ARA disclosure recognizes adolescents' lived experiences and emerging autonomy.

Community violence happens between unrelated individuals, who may or may not know each other, generally outside the home, and often results in assaultive injuries. Community violence interventions can prevent assaultive injuries and assist victims of community violence. Trauma-informed care is foundational to the success of community violence intervention. Place-based environmental interventions can decrease community violence on the population level, and further research and developments are needed in this area. Substance use is a significant barrier to intervention program involvement and greater research and program development is needed to support substance use treatment of those impacted by community violence.

Given recent trends demonstrating increased suicide risk among youth, particularly those from minoritized populations, youth suicide is a major public health concern. Evidence-based practices for the identification and management of youth suicide risk have been developed, yet many challenges exist to implementing them routinely in health care settings. Suggestions for leveraging publicly available resources, gathering input from a range of stakeholders to inform implementation, and enhancing multidisciplinary collaboration are provided with the aim of offering tangible steps toward addressing the youth suicide crisis.

 Video content accompanies this article at http://www.pediatric.theclinics.com.

Firearms are the leading cause of death for US youth, overtaking motor vehicle collisions in 2020. Approximately 65% are due to homicide, 30% are due to suicide, 3.5% are due to unintentional injuries, 2% are undetermined intent, and 0.5% are from legal interventions. In homes with firearms, the likelihood of unintentional death, suicide, and homicide is three to four times higher than those without firearms. Secure storage of firearms, having them locked, unloaded, and separate from ammunition can prevent unintentional firearm injuries.

Child maltreatment is associated with significant morbidity, and prevention is a public health priority. Given evidence of interpersonal and structural racism in child protective service assessment and response, equity must be prioritized for both acute interventions and preventive initiatives aimed at supporting children and their families. Clinicians who care for children are well positioned to support families, and the patient-centered medical home, in collaboration with community-based services, has unique potential as a locus for maltreatment prevention services. Clinicians can advocate for policies that support families and decrease the risk of child maltreatment.

Bullying and School Violence   1153

Daniel J. Flannery, Seth J. Scholer, and Ivette Noriega

Rates of traditional bullying have remained stable (30%) but rates of cyberbullying are increasing rapidly (46% of youth). There are significant long-term physical and mental health consequences of bullying especially for vulnerable youth. Multi-component school-based prevention programs that include caring adults, positive school climate, and supportive services for involved youth can effectively reduce bullying. While bullying has emerged as a legitimate concern, studies of surviving perpetrators to date suggest bullying is not the most significant risk factor of mass school shootings. Pediatricians play a critical role in identification, intervention, awareness, and advocacy.

A Developmentally Informed Approach to Address Mass Firearm Violence   1171

Ashley Sward, Jodi Zik, Amber R. McDonald, Laurel Niep, and Steven Berkowitz

Pediatric medical providers have an important role to play in response to mass gun violence events. Although mass gun violence events are rare, the rate of mass shootings is unfortunately increasing, and such events are shown to have significant and far-reaching psychological impact on children and adolescents. Recommendations from the behavioral health and pediatric fields are consolidated along with developmental considerations to support pediatric provider response in the aftermath of a mass gun violence event. Gun violence prevention strategies are also discussed.

Violence Exposure and Trauma-Informed Care   1183

Michael Arenson and Heather Forkey

Addressing violence in pediatrics requires a working knowledge of trauma-informed care (TIC). TIC weaves together our current understanding of evolution, child development, and human physiology and how these explain common childhood responses to traumatic events. In this article, we describe our current approach to treating childhood trauma in the context of violence. Ultimately, TIC relies on the pediatrician's ability to keep trauma high on their differential diagnosis. TIC leverages a child's natural strengths and biologic processes by (1) scaffolding the patient's relationships to safe, stable, and nurturing adults and (2) strengthening core resilience skills while addressing trauma symptoms when necessary.

Mental Health and Violence in Children and Adolescents   1201

Samaa Kemal, Adaobi Nwabuo, and Jennifer Hoffmann

This article examines the complex interplay between mental health and violence among children. Although children with mental illness are more likely to be victims of violence than perpetrators, this article describes the few mental health conditions associated with increased violent behavior among children. Next, the authors examine the spectrum of mental health sequelae among children following exposure to various forms of violence. Lastly, the authors discuss the underutilization of mental health services in this population and highlight screening and intervention tools available to pediatric clinicians caring for children exposed to violence.

Firearm violence is now the leading cause of youth fatalities in the United States. This article outlines the various ways that entertainment media glorify the use of firearms and how this content can influence youth interest and use of guns. Social media are also increasingly serving as a source of risk for exposure to firearms. Counseling parents about the impact of media exposure to firearms on their children's health, and how to mitigate these risks, can be effective in promoting their children's health and safety.

Given the complexities of youth violence prevention and longstanding violence inequities, advocacy by pediatric clinicians provides a critical voice to represent youth at multiple levels to address the myriad contributors and effects of youth violence. Institutional, community, state, and federal programs, policies, and legislation are required to support a public health approach to the amelioration of youth violence. This article focuses on the role of pediatric clinicians in advocating for youth and families, promoting change within clinical and hospital systems, partnering with communities to advance evidence-informed prevention and intervention, and legislative advocacy to advance violence prevention policy, research, and practice.

PEDIATRIC CLINICS OF NORTH AMERICA

PEDIATRIC CLINICS OF NORTH AMERICA

FORTHCOMING ISSUES

February 2024
Everyday Ethics in the Clinical Practice of
Pediatric and Young Adult Medicine
Margaret R. Moon, Editor

April 2024
Autism Spectrum Disorder
Paul H. Lipkin and Joshua B. Ewen,
Editors

June 2024
Pediatric Planning in Pandemics
Yonca A. Malbora, Steven Selbst and
Erica L. Popovsky, Editors

RECENT ISSUES

October 2023
Pediatric Genetics
Anne Slavotinek, Editor

August 2023
Achieving Child Health Equity
Robert S. Kahn, Monica Mitchell and
Tina L. Cheng, Editors

June 2023
Pediatric Rehabilitation
Mary McMahon and Amy Houtrow,
Editors

Foreword

The Impact of Violence on Child and Adolescent Health

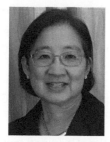

Tina L. Cheng, MD, MPH
Consulting Editor

US child and adolescent all-cause mortality rates have had the largest increase in at least 50 years, rising 20% between 2019 and 2021.[1] These alarming mortality trends among our young began before the pandemic and have been exacerbated by the pandemic. Causes include homicide, motor vehicle injury, and "diseases of despair" of suicide and drug overdose. Firearms have become the number one cause of death for American children aged 0 to 19 years. The child and adolescent firearm death rate in the United States far exceeds other industrialized countries.[2]

Mortalities are much higher among black children and adolescents compared with their white counterparts, and the increase since 2019 disproportionately affects minoritized populations. For example, in 2021, black adolescents aged 10 to 19 years were 20 times more likely to die by homicide than white and Asian American/Pacific Islanders. American Indian/Alaska Native youth had a higher risk of dying from motor vehicle injury. The pandemic laid bare substantial health disparities by race/ethnicity and is expected to reverse at least 10 years of progress in closing the black-white gap in life expectancy.[3]

Violence and health inequity are pervasive in our society, and their impact starts early in the life course. In 1991, when I wrote my public health degree thesis on firearm injury in children, I received critiques that the topic was criminial justice and not public health. We have made progress in recognizing violence as a critical public health issue that requires a public health approach. Preventing violence and buffering its impact are important responsibilities for pediatric clinicians who care about whole child and family

Pediatr Clin N Am 70 (2023) xv–xvi
https://doi.org/10.1016/j.pcl.2023.07.005
0031-3955/23/© 2023 Published by Elsevier Inc.

health. Ensuring health equity is fundamental. This issue provides the needed attention and guidance on major public health issues of our time.

Tina L. Cheng, MD, MPH
Director, Cincinnati Children's Research Foundation
Chief Medical Officer
Cincinnati Children's Hospital Medical Center
3333 Burnet Avenue MLC 3016
Cincinnati, OH 45229-3026, USA

E-mail address:
Tina.cheng@cchmc.org

REFERENCES

1. Woolf SH, Wolf ER, Rivara FP. The new crisis of increasing all-cause mortality in US children and adolescents. JAMA 2023;329(12):975–6. https://doi.org/10.1001/jama.2023.3517. PMID: 36912829.
2. McGough M, Amin K, Panchal N, et al, Kaiser Family Foundation. Child and teen firearm mortality in the US and peer countries. July 2022. Available at: https://www.kff.org/global-health-policy/issue-brief/child-and-teen-firearm-mortality-in-the-u-s-and-peer-countries/. Accessed July 15, 2023.
3. Andrasfay T, Goldman N. Reductions in 2020 US life expectancy due to COVID-19 and the disproportionate impact on the Black and Latino populations. Proc Natl Acad Sci U S A 2021;118(5). https://doi.org/10.1073/pnas.2014746118. p. e2014746118. PMID: 33446511; PMCID: PMC7865122.

Preface

Examining and Addressing Children's Exposure to Violence: The Role of the Pediatric Clinician

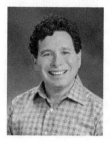   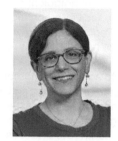

Joel A. Fein, MD, MPH   Megan H. Bair-Merritt, MD, MSCE
Editors

Exposure to violence disrupts a child's health and development more significantly than most other experiences and exposures. This issue of *Pediatric Clinics of North America* is dedicated to helping clinicians identify and support children and families who experience violence in their homes, schools, and neighborhoods. Violence exposure is by nature intersectional, rarely occurring in isolation. Children who are exposed to intimate partner violence are often direct victims of physical or emotional abuse. High levels of community violence can steer parents toward keeping guns in the home to keep the family safe, only to discover that their child's curiosity led to a much more common and tragic outcome of unintentional injury or death. A school-aged child may experience bullying, and graduating to middle or high school places them at higher risk for adolescent relationship abuse. In rare but escalating cases, children are victims of mass shootings. Finally, all of these life experiences can kindle thoughts of suicide. While millions of children across the United States are impacted each year, this public health crisis disproportionately impacts Black and Brown children and other marginalized communities, rooted in historic by historic disinvestment and structural racism.

As many of us can feel in our clinical practices, there has been an uptick in all forms of violence in the past few years, with the United States having the highest rate of child mortality from gun violence across similar nations. In some neighborhoods, the violence literally surrounds our children, and the level of trauma is unimaginable. As a buffer to these exposures, pediatric providers can play an important role as trusted partners for parents and caregivers and can deploy a healing-centered engagement approach to address trauma.

Pediatr Clin N Am 70 (2023) xvii–xviii
https://doi.org/10.1016/j.pcl.2023.07.002
0031-3955/23/© 2023 Published by Elsevier Inc.

pediatric.theclinics.com

Each article in this issue defines a type of violence exposure and offers guidance on how to prevent, or at least mitigate, the impact on our patients and their families. It is squarely within the purview of pediatric clinicians to address these issues and to partner with families to optimize children's physical and mental health, the latter of which is much more often affected as a result, rather than a cause, of violence.

Much of what you will read in this issue emphasizes that it is appropriate, and in fact necessary, to provide anticipatory guidance around sensitive issues, such as childhood trauma, gun safety, and mental illness. Given the time constraints encountered in pediatric practice, many of the sections propose practical strategies to integrate screening and response, as well as technological solutions and partnerships with other disciplines that can more easily facilitate connections to essential resources.

While the content of this issue of *Pediatric Clinics of North America* is largely dedicated to efforts in clinicians' offices or hospital rooms, we also know that many of the most important positive changes need to happen at higher levels. Providers on the front lines are in a powerful position to advocate for greater systems change, including policies that can address the aforementioned disparities. We can use the data and knowledge imparted in many of the sections of this issue, paired with our patients' narratives, to advocate at the local, regional, or national policy levels. Many of the clinicians and researchers who have contributed to this issue have joined in these efforts, and their research and writings have been used by others to support advocacy efforts. On behalf of all of our children, we deeply appreciate the time, effort, and expertise of the section authors for this issue.

Joel A. Fein, MD, MPH
Perelman School of Medicine
University of Pennsylvania
Center for Violence Prevention and Division of Emergency Medicine
Children's Hospital of Philadelphia, Roberts Pediatric Research Building
2716 South Street, 13th Floor
Philadelphia, PA 19146, USA

Megan H. Bair-Merritt, MD, MSCE
Boston Medical Center
Boston University Chobanian & Avedesian School of Medicine
Boston, MA 02118, USA

E-mail addresses:
fein@chop.edu (J.A. Fein)
Megan.Bair-Merritt@bmc.org (M.H. Bair-Merritt)

The Epidemiology of Violence Exposure in Children

Katie A. Donnelly, MD, MPH*, Monika K. Goyal, MD, MSCE

KEYWORDS

- Epidemiology • Violence • Pediatrics • Adverse childhood experiences • Trauma

KEY POINTS

- Violence impacts many American children each day in a variety of forms.
- The COVID-19 pandemic exacerbated the rates of many violence exposures for children.
- The burden of violence unfairly impacts children of color and lesbian, gay, bisexual, transgender, and questioning youth, in large part due to systemic injustice.
- Pediatricians can and must take a role in recognizing, assessing, and treating violence exposure in children.

BACKGROUND

Violence, as defined by the World Health Organization, is "the intentional use of physical force or power, threatened or actual, against oneself, another person, or against a group or community that either results in or has a high likelihood of resulting in injury, death, psychological harm, maldevelopment or deprivation".[1] Violence in all its forms impacts children across the United States each day and is consistently one of the leading causes of child and adolescent mortality.[2] At least 2700 children ages 0 to 18 years died of homicide in 2020, and an estimated additional 160,000 children were injured by violence that same year.[3,4] Research estimates that 60% of all American children will experience at least one form of violence in the home, school, or community each year.[5,6] The different forms of violence experienced by children, such as community violence, intimate partner violence (IPV), and adolescent relationship abuse (ARA), child maltreatment, and bullying, are often interconnected and share similar root causes (**Fig. 1**).[7]

The impact of violence on children, including long-term outcomes, is becoming more and more clear.[8,9] Violence impacts children's physical health through acute

Children's National Hospital, The George Washington University, 111 Michigan Avenue NW, Washington, DC 20010, USA
* Corresponding author.
E-mail address: kdonnell@ChildrensNational.org

Pediatr Clin N Am 70 (2023) 1057–1068
https://doi.org/10.1016/j.pcl.2023.06.005
0031-3955/23/© 2023 Elsevier Inc. All rights reserved.

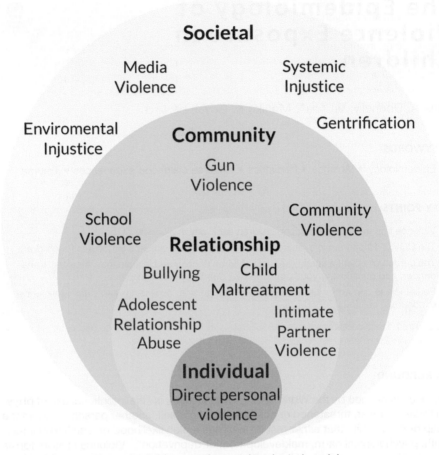

Fig. 1. Violence exposure in children on the social ecological model.

biologic responses, like raising cortisol levels and disrupting sleep.[10] It can also deter behaviors that promote health, such as physical activity, due to safety concerns.[11,12] Exposure to violence of any kind also affects a child's mental health, contributing to the development of post-traumatic stress disorder, anxiety, and depression. Exposure to violence in childhood and adolescence can also have significant effects on the developing brain, particularly in infants and young children.[13] Unfortunately, experiencing violence as a child can sometimes lead to the perpetration of violence and involvement with criminal justice in the future. This "cycle of violence" has been evident in varying forms of violence exposure and across multiple communities.[14–17]

TYPES OF VIOLENCE EXPERIENCED BY CHILDREN
Intimate Partner Violence

IPV is abuse or aggression that occurs in a current or prior romantic relationship and can include multiple forms, such as physical violence, sexual violence, stalking, psychological aggression, financial coercion, cyber abuse/bullying, and isolation.[18] IPV is common, with an estimated 15.5 million children exposed to IPV each year through their parents' and caregivers' relationships.[19] Lifetime prevalence of IPV is high regardless of gender, with 47.3% of women and 44.2% of men reporting any sexual violence, physical violence, or stalking.[20] Women of color report higher rates of IPV than those who identify as White.[21,22] Marginalized communities, such as communities of color, immigrants, those living in poverty, sexual and gender diverse persons, and other communities, may experience IPV differently and may be more or less likely to report it for a variety of reasons.[23] This topic is explored in greater detail in the next article in this volume. During the COVID-19 pandemic, there was an increase in both the prevalence and severity of IPV, with having a toddler in the home being a significant risk factor for experiencing IPV.[24]

Adolescent Relationship Abuse

ARA, often called teen dating violence, refers to IPV that occurs directly in the relationship of the adolescent. ARA is common, with 1 in 12 adolescents experiencing physical dating violence, and another 1 in 12 experiencing sexual dating violence.[25] Among adolescents who had dated in the past year, 69% reported lifetime ARA victimization and 63% reported ARA perpetration.[26] Though ARA can affect all teenagers, female and lesbian, gay, bisexual, transgender, and questioning (LGBTQ) teenagers are more likely to experience all forms of ARA when compared with heterosexual peers (physical 43% vs 29%, psychological 59% vs 46%, cyber dating abuse 37% vs 26%, sexual coercion 23 vs 12%).[27,28] Adolescents are more likely to experience ARA online as well, through email, text, or social media sites.[29,30] ARA can also turn fatal, with 7% of adolescent homicides committed by intimate partners.[31] During the COVID-19 pandemic, rates of ARA stayed similar or even improved compared with pre-pandemic rates, perhaps due to school closures and social distancing.[32]

Community Violence

Community violence is violence that occurs between unrelated individuals who may or may not know each other, outside of the home.[33] Community violence is direct (personal victimization) or indirect (witnessing violence), with children more likely to experience indirect community violence.[33] Indirect violence exposure can include seeing violent acts, watching someone be threatened, or hearing gunshots.[34] Witnessing physical violence in communities is high, with 44% to 82% of children reporting seeing a non-relation be slapped, hit, or punched.[33] About 13% of children in the United States have seen someone threatened with a weapon in their communities and 41% have experienced indirect community gun violence, such as hearing gunshots.[35,36] Boys are more likely to experience direct community violence than girls and children of color are more likely to live in neighborhoods with high exposure to community violence.[31,33] Exposure to community violence can have significant effects on children's physical and mental health, as well as school performance.[37-39] During the COVID-19 pandemic, community violence increased in some communities, especially racial and ethnic minoritized communities, as measured by emergency department visits for all violent injuries.[40-42]

Gun Violence

Since 2019, gun violence, whether through homicide or suicide or accident, has been identified as the number one cause of death in children in the United States, overtaking motor vehicle accidents.[43] Per the Gun Violence Archive, more than 1600 children ages 0 to 17 years were killed by guns in 2022 and more than 4500 were injured.[44] The United States accounts for more than 90% of pediatric gun fatalities among similar peer countries.[45] Gun violence disproportionately impacts children of color, especially Black youth, who are significantly more likely to die of gun assaults than their White peers; firearms have been the leading cause of death in Black children since 2001.[46] Suicide by firearm is more common among White children, though rates are also rising among Black young adults.[47] Mass shootings, especially in schools, continue to be a uniquely American problem with upward trends in rates of mass shootings over the past 5 years.[48] During the COVID-19 pandemic, both children injured and killed by firearms and those exposed to firearm violence increased.[49–51] The racial disparity in gunshot injuries dramatically increased during the pandemic, with a 4 fold increase for Black compared with White children.[52] Firearm purchases also increased during the pandemic, leading to a large number of new families and children potentially exposed to firearms.[53]

Bullying

Bullying is defined as "any unwanted aggressive behavior by a youth or group of youths that are not siblings or current dating partners that involves an observed or perceived power imbalance that is repeated".[54] Bullying is physical, verbal, relational, or cause damage to the property of the victim. Bullying is associated with other violent behaviors and exposures and should not be thought of as just a normal part of childhood.[55,56] Bullying is unequally experienced, with LGBTQ children experiencing significantly more bullying than their heterosexual peers.[57] Bullying rates in American youth have stayed steady over the past 25 years, with about 20% of youth reporting bullying on school grounds.[25] Cyberbullying, or bullying that occurs online through email or social media, has risen as adolescents engage more with social media.[58] Cyberbullying can consist of offensive name-calling, spreading false rumors, receiving explicit images, stalking, physical threats, or having explicit images of themselves shared without their consent, with 46% of 13 to 17 year olds reporting at least one of those examples.[59] The COVID-19 pandemic seemed to disrupt both in person and cyberbullying as it prevented children from going to school, yet rates have begun to rise to prepandemic levels as children returned to school.[60]

Child Maltreatment

Child maltreatment, or child abuse and neglect, is defined as "any act or series of acts of commission or omission by a parent, caregiver or another person in a custodial role that results in harm, potential for harm or threat of harm to a child."[61] This can encompass physical abuse, sexual abuse, emotional abuse, or neglect. At least 1 in 7 children experience child maltreatment each year in the United States and there have been no significant changes in the rate of child maltreatment.[62] About one-third of all children will experience a child protective services (CPS) investigation before the age of 18 years, with the percentage being highest for Black children (53%).[63] This disparity in CPS investigations is likely due to both intrapersonal racism or individual biases and systemic racism that leads to unjust policies and practices.[64,65] These disparities are discussed in detail in Tolliver and colleagues' article, "Child Maltreatment," in this issue. During the COVID-19 pandemic, emergency department visits for child abuse evaluations decreased but hospitalizations stayed the same or even rose.[66] Some have hypothesized that less severe forms of child abuse that might have been identified by other mandated reporters, like school officials or daycare staff, were not reported due to lockdowns closing these institutions.

Media Violence

Exposure to media violence, which includes real or simulated violence in television, music, social media, and video games, is harmful to children's health and is associated with increased aggressive behaviors and fears.[67] School age children view media about 5 hours each day, while teenagers jump up to 7.5 hours, not including school-work or homework, though this time does include multi-tasking, such as listening to YouTube videos while getting ready in the morning.[68] Most young people see some form of violence in the media they consume each day.[69] More research is needed, however, to further investigate the media violence to which children are currently exposed, especially with new social media applications.[69] During the COVID-19 pandemic, media use among children and teens increased, which likely increased the amount of media violence those children were exposed to as well.[70] The influence of media violence on children will be discussed in the Michael Arenson and Heather Forkey's article, "Violence Exposure and Trauma-Informed Care," in this issue on Media Exposure and Violence.

DISCUSSION
Inequities of Pediatric Violence Exposure

One cannot fully discuss the epidemiology of violence without exploring the forces that drive the data. Exposure to violence and its impact are disproportionately distributed, with children of color and LGBTQ children often experiencing more violence than White, heterosexual peers.[27,50,51–70] For instance, Black and Hispanic youth report higher rates of ARA compared with White peers, and rates are even higher among those with intersectional identities (eg, sex or gender).[71–73] This disparity is most likely due to the systemic injustices that continue in the places where we work, live, and play. Minoritized populations are disproportionately exposed to poverty, racism, limited educational and occupational opportunities, and other aspects of social and economic disadvantages that contribute to violence.[74,75] These disparities are sustained due to the persistence of these societal disadvantages, and may even be exacerbated because exposure to childhood trauma and adversity is a risk factor for intergenerational violence victimization and perpetration.[76]

One reason these inequities exist is due to the concentration of poverty and minoritized populations in segregated neighborhoods. These neighborhoods were created out of the 1950s practice of redlining by the federal government's Home Owner's Loan Corporation, denying capital investment to "high-risk" neighborhoods, the majority of which were populated by low-income and minoritized communities.[77] Though redlining is no longer allowed, neighborhoods remain segregated as a result of those policies.[77] Firearm shootings are higher in neighborhoods that had been redlined, even when controlling for other confounders.[78] Redlining has been associated with environmental injustice, with affected neighborhoods having higher levels of lead and air pollution and less green space and parks.[79–81] Decades of racist policies have led to unsafe streets, not just from violence itself, but also just to walk as a pedestrian or drive a car.[82]

Yet attempts to rectify the effects of redlining may also have an impact on minoritized communities, specifically through gentrification. Gentrification involves neighborhoods that have historically experienced disinvestment and economic decline then experiencing reinvestment, with a higher socioeconomic status population migrating into that neighborhood.[83] As neighborhoods gentrify, violent incidents like firearm shootings shift to non-gentrified areas, likely further impacting displaced families of color.[84] Though there are limited data on the effects of gentrification on children, there is evidence that children experiencing gentrification of their neighborhood have increases in diagnoses of anxiety or depression.[85] Gentrification often increases the policing of the neighborhood as well to protect property and wealth.[86] Subsequent over-policing of Black communities leads to greater inequities in the justice system. Youth of color are more likely to die due to legal intervention than non-Hispanic White youth.[87] Being stopped by the police is a stronger predictor of post-traumatic stress disorder among Black college students than experiencing direct victimization by community violence.[88] Police presence in hospitals can lead to physical and mental health effects and provider mistrust.[89]

Health care's Role in Addressing Pediatric Violence Exposure

As pediatricians, we have a unique relationship with children and families who have been exposed to violence. The American Academy of Pediatrics has a comprehensive policy statement on the role of pediatricians in preventing youth violence, including being active in the domains of clinical care, advocacy, education, and research.[90] Families impacted by violence may not trust law enforcement or government help but may feel comfortable discussing their trauma with a medical provider.[91] We may even take care of these patients when they are acutely injured by violence. Therefore, it is imperative that we are ready to assess our patients for violence exposure and that we are familiar with community support resources.

Understanding the scope of violence and its impact on patients is a critical component of our practice as pediatricians. A previous way of measuring violence and trauma exposure in children has been by tracking the number of adverse childhood experiences (ACEs) that a child has experienced.[92] Yet these scores do not capture the depth or impact of trauma or violence on an individual or how different ACEs have differential impacts when combined. Additionally, the 10 original ACEs do not include other forms of violence that have been recognized as having impacts on long-term health, such as racism and discrimination, community violence, sexual assault, school violence, or bullying.[93] Therefore, ACE scores are less favored as a screening tool and should not be used to predict individual-level impact on a single patient.[94] Instead, there is a rising movement to provide universal information and resources.[95,96] This moves providers away from needing a disclosure to offer education and supports for those who have experienced violence. It is also important for pediatricians to understand the need to prevent retraumatization when patients seek medical care for any reason, not just violent injury. One way to accomplish this is to practice trauma-informed care (TIC), that is to assess, recognize, and respond to the effects of traumatic stress on our patients and families.[97,98] TIC practices will be discussed in greater detail in the study on "Violence Exposure and Trauma-Informed Care".

An additional role for pediatricians, given the inequities outlined above, is advocacy. Whether it means fighting for a new program to address violence, obtaining a grant to research these exposures, or making our health care systems more equitable and just, we can all find ways to advocate for our patients and families who have experienced and are experiencing violence.[99] We also must educate future pediatricians on how to incorporate advocacy into their daily practice.[100] We can consider how we can expand the reach of our advocacy beyond the walls into our hospitals and clinics, through both community and governmental involvement. It is only through this continued effort that we will be able to stem the effects of violence on our patients.

SUMMARY

Exposure to violence remains a significant issue for children in the United States. The COVID-19 pandemic exacerbated many of these exposures. Violence unequally impacts children of color and LGBTQ youth. Pediatricians can and must continue to advocate and intervene to decrease pediatric violence exposure and its effects.

CLINICS CARE POINTS

- Remember that violence, in all its forms, affects many children in your practice.
- Universal screening and provision of resources can help support children and families who have experienced violence.

DISCLOSURE

Dr K.A. Donnelly receives funding from the Office of Victim Services and Justice Grants (OVSJG) in Washington, DC as the medical director for the Youth Violence Intervention Program at Children's National.

REFERENCES

1. Krug EG, Dahlberg LL, Mercy JA, et al. World report on violence and health. Geneva: World Health Organization; 2002.
2. Heron M. National Vital Statistics Reports. Deaths: Leading Causes for 2019; 2021. Available at: https://www.cdc.gov/nchs/data/nvsr/nvsr70/nvsr70-09-508. pdf. Accessed April 14, 2023.
3. Centers for Disease Control and Prevention. WISQARS Fatal Injury Data Visualization. Available at: https://wisqars-viz.cdc.gov:8006/explore-data/home. Accessed April 24, 20223.
4. Centers for Diseases Control and Prevention. Injury - WISQARS Non-fatal Injury Data Visualizaiton. Available at: https://wisqars-viz.cdc.gov:8006/explore-data/ home. Accessed April 24, 2023.
5. Finkelhor D, Turner H, Ormrod R, et al. Children's exposure to violence: a comprehensive national survey. Juvenile Justice Bulletin 2009. https://doi.org/ 10.1016/0278-2391(95)90744-0.
6. Finkelhor D, Turner HA, Shattuck A, et al. Violence, crime, and abuse exposure in a national sample of children and youth an update. JAMA Pediatr 2013; 167(7). https://doi.org/10.1001/jamapediatrics.2013.42.
7. Wilkins N, Tsao B, Hertz M, et al. Connecting the Dots: An Overview of the Links Among Multiple Forms of Violence.; 2014. Available at: https://www.cdc.gov/ violenceprevention/about/connectingthedots.html. Accessed November 2, 2022.
8. Moffitt TE, Arseneault L, Danese A, et al. Childhood exposure to violence and lifelong health: clinical intervention science and stress-biology research join forces. Dev Psychopathol 2013;25(4):1619–34.
9. de Bellis MD, Zisk A. The biological effects of childhood trauma. Child Adolesc Psychiatr Clin N Am 2014;23(2):185–222.
10. Heissel JA, Sharkey PT, Torrats-Espinosa G, et al. Violence and vigilance: the acute effects of community violent crime on sleep and cortisol. Child Dev 2018;89(4):e323–31.
11. Gómez JE, Johnson BA, Selva M, et al. Violent crime and outdoor physical activity among inner-city youth. Prev Med 2004;39(5):876–81.
12. Molnar BE, Gortmaker SL, Bull FC, et al. Unsafe to play? Neighborhood disorder and lack of safety predict reduced physical activity among urban children and adolescents. Am J Health Promot 2004;18(5):378–86.
13. Tomaszewski E, editor. National academies of sciences the neurocognitive and psychosocial impacts of violence and trauma. Washington, DC: National Academies Press; 2018. https://doi.org/10.17226/25077.

14. Bingenheimer JB, Brennan RT, Earls FJ. Sociology: Firearm violence exposure and serious violent behavior. Science (1979) 2005;308(5726):1323–6.

15. Gömez AM. Testing the cycle of violence hypothesis: child abuse and adolescent dating violence as predictors of intimate partner violence in young adulthood. Youth Soc 2011;43(1):171–92.

16. Ma J, Grogan-Kaylor A, Delva J. Behavior problems among adolescents exposed to family and community violence in chile. Fam Relat 2016;65(3): 502–16.

17. Turanovic JJ, Pratt TC. Consequences of violent victimization for native american youth in early adulthood. J Youth Adolesc 2017;46(6):1333–50.

18. Stylianou AM. Economic abuse within intimate partner violence: a review of the literature. Violence Vict 2018;33(1):3–22.

19. McDonald R, Jouriles EN, Ramisetty-Mikler S, et al. Estimating the number of American children living in partner-violent families. J Fam Psychol 2006;20(1): 137–42.

20. Centers for Disease Control and Prevention The National Intimate Partner and Sexual Violence Survey: 2016/2017 Report on Intimate Partner Violence.; 2016. Available at: https://www.cdc.gov/violenceprevention/pdf/nisvs/nisvsreportonipv_2022.pdf. Accessed April 20, 2023.

21. Schafer J, Caetano R, Clark CL. Rates of intimate partner violence in the United States. Am J Public Health 1998;88(11). https://doi.org/10.2105/AJPH.88.11.1702.

22. Stockman JK, Hayashi H, Campbell JC. Intimate partner violence and its health impact on disproportionately affected populations, including minorities and impoverished groups. J Womens Health 2015;24(1):62–79.

23. Ragavan MI, Thomas KA, Fulambarker A, et al. Exploring the needs and lived experiences of racial and ethnic minority domestic violence survivors through community-based participatory research: a systematic review. Trauma Violence Abuse 2020;21(5):946–63.

24. Peitzmeier SM, Fedina L, Ashwell L, et al. Increases in intimate partner violence during COVID-19: prevalence and correlates. J Interpers Violence 2022; 37(21–22):NP20482–512.

25. Centers for Disease Control. Youth Risk Behavior Surveillance System: Adolescent and School Health | CDC. Available at: https://www.cdc.gov/healthyyouth/data/yrbs/index.htm. Accessed April 23, 2022.

26. Taylor BG, Mumford EA. A national descriptive portrait of adolescent relationship abuse: results from the national survey on teen relationships and intimate violence. J Interpers Violence 2016;31(6):963–88.

27. Dank M, Lachman P, Zweig JM, et al. Dating violence experiences of lesbian, gay, bisexual, and transgender youth. J Youth Adolesc 2014;43(5):846–57.

28. Breiding MJ. Prevalence and characteristics of sexual violence, stalking, and intimate partner violence victimization - National intimate partner and sexual violence survey, United States, 2011. Am J Public Health 2015;105(4):e11–2.

29. Zweig J, Dank M. Teen Dating Abuse and Harassment in the Digital World.; 2013. Available at: https://www.urban.org/sites/default/files/publication/23326/412750-Teen-Dating-Abuse-and-Harassment-in-the-Digital-World.PDF. Accessed January 22, 2023.

30. Ortega-Barón J, Montiel I, Machimbarrena JM, et al. Epidemiology of Cyber dating abuse victimization in adolescence and its relationship with health-related quality of life: a longitudinal study. Youth Soc 2022;54(5):711–29.

31. Adhia A, Kernic MA, Hemenway D, et al. Intimate partner homicide of adolescents. JAMA Pediatr 2019;173(6):571–7.
32. Krause KH, DeGue S, Kilmer G, et al. Prevalence and correlates of non-dating sexual violence, sexual dating violence, and physical dating violence victimization among U.S. High School Students during the COVID-19 pandemic: adolescent behaviors and experiences survey, United States, 2021. J Interpers Violence 2022. https://doi.org/10.1177/08862605221140038.
33. Stein BD, Jaycox LH, Kataoka S, et al. Prevalence of child and adolescent exposure to community violence. Clin Child Fam Psychol Rev 2003;6(4):247–64.
34. Thompson R, Proctor LJ, Weisbart C, et al. Children's self-reports about violence exposure: an examination of the things i have seen and heard scale. Am J Orthopsychiatry 2007;77(3):454–66.
35. Mitchell KJ, Hamby SL, Turner HA, et al. Weapon involvement in the victimization of children. Pediatrics 2015;136(1):10–7.
36. Mitchell KJ, Jones LM, Turner HA, et al. Understanding the impact of seeing gun violence and hearing gunshots in public places: findings from the youth firearm risk and safety study. J Interpers Violence 2021;36(17–18). https://doi.org/10.1177/0886260519853393.
37. Wright AW, Austin M, Booth C, et al. Exposure to community violence and physical health outcomes in youth: a systematic review. J Pediatr Psychol 2016;42(4):jsw088.
38. Matthay EC, Farkas K, Skeem J, et al. Exposure to community violence and self-harm in California. Epidemiology 2018;29(5):697–706.
39. Koposov R, Isaksson J, Vermeiren R, et al. Community violence exposure and school functioning in youth: cross-country and gender perspectives. Front Public Health 2021;9:1058.
40. O'Neill KM, Dodington J, Gawel M, et al. The effect of the COVID-19 pandemic on community violence in Connecticut. Am J Surg 2022. https://doi.org/10.1016/j.amjsurg.2022.10.004.
41. Beiter K, Danos D, Conrad E, et al. The COVID-19 pandemic and associated increases in experiences of assault violence among black men with low socioeconomic status living in Louisiana. Heliyon 2022;8(7):e09974.
42. Vasan A, Mitchell HK, Fein JA, et al. Association of neighborhood gun violence with mental health-related pediatric emergency department utilization. JAMA Pediatr 2021 Dec 1;175(12):1244–51.
43. Goldstick JE, Cunningham RM, Carter PM. Current causes of death in children and adolescents in the United States. N Engl J Med 2022;386(20):1955–6.
44. Gun Violence Archive. Available at: https://www.gunviolencearchive.org/. Accessed April 23, 2023.
45. Grinshteyn E, Hemenway D. Violent death rates in the US compared to those of the other high-income countries, 2015. Prev Med 2019;123:20–6.
46. Andrews AL, Killings X, Oddo ER, et al. Pediatric firearm injury mortality epidemiology. Pediatrics 2022;149(3). https://doi.org/10.1542/PEDS.2021-052739/184887.
47. Kaplan MS, Mueller-Williams AC, Goldman-Mellor S, et al. Changing trends in suicide mortality and firearm involvement among black young adults in the United States, 1999–2019. Arch Suicide Res 2022. https://doi.org/10.1080/13811118.2022.2098889.
48. Katsiyannis A, Rapa LJ, Whitford DK, et al. An examination of US school mass shootings, 2017–2022: findings and implications. Adv Neurodev Disord 2022. https://doi.org/10.1007/s41252-022-00277-3.

49. Bernardin ME, Clukies L, Gu H, et al. COVID-19 pandemic effects on the epidemiology and mortality of pediatric firearm injuries; a single center study. J Pediatr Surg 2022. https://doi.org/10.1016/j.jpedsurg.2022.10.007.

50. Martin R, Rajan S, Shareef F, et al. Racial disparities in child exposure to firearm violence before and during COVID-19. Am J Prev Med 2022;63(2):204–12.

51. Cohen JS, Donnelly K, Patel SJ, et al. Firearms injuries involving young children in the United States during the COVID-19 pandemic. Pediatrics 2021;148(1). https://doi.org/10.1542/peds.2020-042697.

52. Jay J, Martin R, Patel M, et al. Analyzing child firearm assault injuries by race and ethnicity during the COVID-19 pandemic in 4 major US cities. JAMA Netw Open 2023;6(3):e233125.

53. Miller M, Zhang W, Azrael D. Firearm purchasing during the COVID-19 pandemic: results from the 2021 national firearms survey. Ann Intern Med 2022;175(2):219–25.

54. Fast Fact: Preventing Bullying |Violence Prevention|Injury Center|CDC. Available at: https://www.cdc.gov/violenceprevention/youthviolence/bullyingresearch/fastfact.html. Accessed January 25, 2023.

55. Nansel TR, Ovevpeck MD, Haynie DL, et al. Relationships between bullying and violence among US youth. Arch Pediatr Adolesc Med 2003;157(4):348–53.

56. Kreski NT, Chen Q, Olfson M, et al. Experiences of online bullying and offline violence-related behaviors among a nationally representative sample of <scp>US</scp> adolescents, 2011 to 2019. J Sch Health 2022;92(4):376–86.

57. Earnshaw VA, Reisner SL, Juvonen J, et al. LGBTQ bullying: translating research to action in pediatrics. Pediatrics 2017;140(4).

58. Kennedy RS. Bullying Trends in the United States: A Meta-Regression. Trauma Violence Abuse 2021;22(4):914–27.

59. Teens and Cyberbullying 2022 | Pew Research Center. Available at: https://www.pewresearch.org/internet/2022/12/15/teens-and-cyberbullying-2022/. Accessed April 23, 2023.

60. Bacher-Hicks A., Goodman J., Green J.G., & Holt M.K. The COVID-19 pandemic disrupted both school bullying and cyberbullying. *Am Econ Rev: Insights*, 4(3), 2020, 353-370.

61. Leeb RT, Paulozzi LJ, Melanson C, et al. Child maltreatment surveillance: Uniform Definitions for Public Health and Recommended Data Elements Version 1.0.; 2008.

62. Finkelhor D, Turner HA, Shattuck A, et al. Prevalence of childhood exposure to violence, crime, and abuse: Results from the National Survey of Children's Exposure to Violence. JAMA Pediatr 2015;169(8):746–54.

63. Kim H, Wildeman C, Jonson-Reid M, et al. Lifetime prevalence of investigating child maltreatment among US children. Am J Public Health 2017;107(2):274–80.

64. Thomas MMC, Waldfogel J, Williams OF. Inequities in child protective services contact between black and white children. Child Maltreat 2023;28(1):42–54.

65. Dettlaff AJ, Boyd R. Racial disproportionality and disparities in the child welfare system: why do they exist, and what can be done to address them? Ann Am Acad Pol Soc Sci 2020;692(1):253–74.

66. Swedo E, Idaikkadar N, Leemis R, et al. Trends in U.S. Emergency department visits related to suspected or confirmed child abuse and neglect among children and adolescents aged <18 years before and during the COVID-19 pandemic — United States, January 2019–September 2020. MMWR Morb Mortal Wkly Rep 2020;69(49):1841–7.

67. Fuld GL, Mulligan DA, Altmann TR, et al. Policy statement - Media violence. Pediatrics 2009;124(5):1495–503.
68. Common Sense Media. The Common Sense Census: Media Use by Tweens and Teens | Common Sense Media. Published 2019. Available at: https://www.commonsensemedia.org/research/the-common-sense-census-media-use-by-tweens-and-teens-2019. Accessed February 19, 2023.
69. Common Sense Media. Media and Violence: An Analysis of Current Research.; 2013. Available at: https://www.commonsensemedia.org/sites/default/files/research/report/media-and-violence-research-brief-2013.pdf. Accessed February 19, 2023.
70. Kroshus E, Tandon PS, Zhou C, et al. Problematic child media use during the COVID-19 pandemic. Pediatrics 2022;150(3). https://doi.org/10.1542/peds.2021-055190.
71. Whitton SW, Lawlace M, Dyar C, et al. Exploring mechanisms of racial disparities in intimate partner violence among sexual and gender minorities assigned female at birth. Cultur Divers Ethnic Minor Psychol 2021;27(4):602–12.
72. Steele SM, Everett BG, Hughes TL. Influence of perceived femininity, masculinity, race/ethnicity, and socioeconomic status on intimate partner violence among sexual-minority women. J Interpers Violence 2020;35(1–2):453–75.
73. Reuter TR, Newcomb ME, Whitton SW, et al. Intimate partner violence victimization in LGBT young adults: demographic differences and associations with health behaviors. Psychol Violence 2017;7(1):101–9.
74. Wilson WJ. The truly disadvantaged: the inner city, the underclass, and public policy. 2nd edition. Chicago: University of Chicago Press; 2012.
75. Sheats KJ, Irving SM, Mercy JA, et al. Violence-related disparities experienced by black youth and young adults: opportunities for prevention. Am J Prev Med 2018;55(4):462–9.
76. Lansford JE, Miller-Johnson S, Berlin LJ, et al. Early physical abuse and later violent delinquency: a prospective longitudinal study. Child Maltreat 2007;12(3):233–45.
77. Mitchell B., Franco J., HOLC "REDLINING" MAPS: the persistent structure of segregation and economic inequality. Available at: www.ncrc.org. Accessed May 2, 2023.
78. Poulson M, Neufeld MY, Dechert T, et al. Historic redlining, structural racism, and firearm violence: a structural equation modeling approach. The Lancet Regional Health - Americas 2021;3. https://doi.org/10.1016/j.lana.2021.100052.
79. Nardone A, Rudolph KE, Morello-Frosch R, et al. Redlines and greenspace: the relationship between historical redlining and 2010 greenspace across the United States. Environ Health Perspect 2021;129(1):1–9.
80. Karp RJ. Redlining and lead poisoning: causes and consequences. J Health Care Poor Underserved 2023;34(1):431–46.
81. Lane HM, Morello-Frosch R, Marshall JD, et al. Historical redlining is associated with present-day air pollution disparities in U.S. Cities. Environ Sci Technol Lett 2022;9(4):345–50.
82. Hauptman M, Bruccoleri R, Woolf AD. An update on childhood lead poisoning. Clin Pediatr Emerg Med 2017;18(3):181–92.
83. Schnake-Mahl AS, Jahn JL, Subramanian Sv, et al. Gentrification, neighborhood change, and population health: a systematic review. J Urban Health 2020;97(1):1.
84. Scantling D, Orji W, Hatchimonji J, et al. Firearm violence, access to care, and gentrification. Ann Surg 2021;274(2):209–17.

85. Dragan KL, Ellen IG, Glied SA. Gentrification and the health of low-income children in New York city. Health Aff 2019;38(9):1425–32.

86. Beck B. Policing gentrification: stops and low–level arrests during demographic change and real estate reinvestment. City Community 2020;19(1):245–72.

87. Badolato GM, Boyle MD, McCarter R, et al. Racial and ethnic disparities in firearm-related pediatric deaths related to legal intervention. Pediatrics 2020; 146(6). https://doi.org/10.1542/peds.2020-015917.

88. Lewis MW, Wu L. Exposure to community violence versus overpolicing and PTSD among African American university students. J Hum Behav Soc Environ 2021;31(8):1026–39.

89. Gallen K, Sonnenberg J, Loughran C, et al. Health effects of policing in hospitals: a narrative review. J Racial Ethn Health Disparities 2022. https://doi.org/10.1007/s40615-022-01275-w.

90. Smith GA, Baum CR, Dowd MD, et al. Policy statement - role of the pediatrician in youth violence prevention. Pediatrics 2009;124(1):393–402.

91. Horowitz K, McKay M, Marshall R. Community violence and urban families: experiences, effects, and directions for intervention. Am J Orthopsychiatry 2005; 75(3):356–68.

92. Felitti VJ, Anda RF, Nordenberg D, et al. Relationship of childhood abuse and household dysfunction to many of the leading causes of death in adults: The adverse childhood experiences (ACE) study. Am J Prev Med 1998;14(4): 245–58.

93. Amaya-Jackson L., Absher L.E., Gerrity E.T., et al., Beyond the ACE Score: Perspectives from the NCTSN on Child Trauma and Adversity Screening and Impact.; 2021. Available at: www.NCTSN.org. Accessed May 4, 2023.

94. Anda RF, Porter LE, Brown DW. Inside the adverse childhood experience score: strengths, limitations, and misapplications. Am J Prev Med 2020;59(2):293–5.

95. Miller E, McCaw B. Intimate partner violence. N Engl J Med 2019;380(9):850–7. https://doi.org/10.1056/NEJMra1807166. Ropper AH.

96. Ragavan MI, Garcia R, Berger RP, et al. Supporting intimate partner violence survivors and their children during the COVID-19 pandemic. Pediatrics 2020; 146(3). https://doi.org/10.1542/PEDS.2020-1276.

97. Forkey H, Szilagyi M, Kelly ET, et al. Trauma-informed care. Pediatrics 2021; 148(2). https://doi.org/10.1542/peds.2021-052580.

98. Marsac ML, Kassam-Adams N, Hildenbrand AK, et al. Implementing a trauma-informed approach in pediatric health care networks. JAMA Pediatr 2016; 170(1):70–7.

99. Camero K, Javier JR. Community advocacy in pediatric practice: perspectives from the field. Pediatr Clin North Am 2023;70(1):43–51.

100. Dodson NA, Talib HJ, Gao Q, et al. Pediatricians as child health advocates: the role of advocacy education. Health Promot Pract 2021;22(1):13–7. https://doi.org/10.1177/1524839920931494.

Supporting Intimate Partner Violence Survivors and Their Children in Pediatric Healthcare Settings

Maya I. Ragavan, MD, MPH, MS[a],*, Ashlee Murray, MD, MPH[b]

KEYWORDS

- Intimate partner violence • Domestic violence • Pediatric health care
- Healing-centered engagement • Victim services agencies
- Community-medical partnerships

KEY POINTS

- Intimate partner violence (IPV) is a pervasive public health epidemic that influences child health and thriving. In this article, we discuss how pediatric health-care providers and systems can create healing-centered spaces to support IPV survivors and their children.
- We review the use of universal education and resource provision to share information about IPV during all clinical encounters as a healing-centered alternative to screening.
- We also review how to support survivors who may share experiences of IPV, focused on validation, affirmation, and connection to resources. Community-medical partnership development to collaborate with victim services agencies is discussed as are evidenced-based IPV training.

In April 2021, as coronavirus disease 2019 (COVID-19) vaccination efforts were underway, a parent and her 2 children came to a pediatric primary care clinic for worsening enuresis. Privately, the parent shared that they were experiencing compounding stressors since the pandemic began, due to her expartner and coparent. He tried to keep her children away from her, stating that her job as a nursing assistant put her at high risk of being infected with COVID-19 and intermittently shut off her cellphone service. She was hesitant to reach out to services because she was not sure if what was happening constituted as "abuse" and did not know to whom to turn. Together, we called a local victim services agency, who provided legal services and

[a] Division of General Academic Pediatrics, University of Pittsburgh and UPMC Children's Hospital of Pittsburgh, 3414 Fifth Avenue, Pittsburgh, PA 15213, USA; [b] Division of Pediatric Emergency Medicine, Children's Hospital of Pennsylvania, 3401 Civic Center Boulevard, Philadelphia, PA 19104, USA
* Corresponding author.
E-mail address: ragavanm@chp.edu

Pediatr Clin N Am 70 (2023) 1069–1086
https://doi.org/10.1016/j.pcl.2023.06.016
0031-3955/23/© 2023 Elsevier Inc. All rights reserved.

supports, as well as helped her procure her own cellular phone. At a follow-up visit, she noted that her partner was now trying to use her diagnosis of depression to get custody of her children but felt well supported by the victim services agency.

Intimate partner violence (IPV) is a pervasive public health epidemic causing health impacts across the life span. The National Intimate Partner and Sexual Violence Survey found that nearly 47% of women and 44% of men have experienced sexual violence, physical violence, and/or stalking at some point in their lives.[1] For women, 27% first experienced IPV before the age of 18, and of those reporting IPV, 1 in 3 was injured and 1 in 8 needed medical care.[1] Historically, IPV research has been gender binary; important emerging work is showing that gender diverse people (sex assigned at birth does not match gender, such as transgender and gender nonbinary) are more likely to experience IPV, rooted in transphobia, genderism, and homophobia.[2,3] Finally, data show that 1 in 5 children are exposed to IPV, and this number increases to 1 in 4 during adolescence[4] with even higher prevalence for youth experiencing marginalization.[5] Pediatric clinicians have a responsibility and opportunity to support IPV survivors and their children using healing-centered approaches.[6,7]

INTIMATE PARTNER VIOLENCE IS ROOTED IN POWER AND CONTROL

Fundamentally, IPV is rooted in power and control, where an abusive partner uses different behaviors and tactics to control, discredit, manipulate, or assert power over their partner. Power and control behaviors may occur in a variety of ways including through isolation, threats, physical or sexual violence, economic or financial coercion (eg, ruining someone's credit), spiritual abuse, immigration-related abuse, among others.[8–10] For example, during the COVID-19 pandemic, IPV survivors reported that partners took their stimulus checks, tried to limit their health-care access, and would turn off Wi-Fi and cellular technology thereby isolating them during shelter-in-place orders.[11–13] Important to pediatrics is use of children (especially child custody) to manipulate or control IPV survivors.[14,15] IPV can also manifest *within* pediatric health-care settings, by abusive partners controlling medical decision, manipulating appointment times, or stalking through use of patient portals.[16]

STRUCTURAL OPPRESSIONS INFLUENCING INTIMATE PARTNER VIOLENCE SURVIVORS FROM MARGINALIZED COMMUNITIES

IPV affects all communities; however, survivors from marginalized communities, including those identifying as people of color (Black, Indigenous, Latine [a gender-neutral alternative to Latino/a or Hispanic], Asian, Pacific Islander, and Multiracial), sexual and gender diverse, immigrants and refugees, non-English speaking, or survivors living in poverty or with disabilities may be uniquely affected by IPV.[17] The lived experiences of IPV survivors from marginalized communities can be situated within intersectionality theory, which describes that social category (ie, race, immigration status, language, and socioeconomic status) intersect at the microlevel to affect individual experiences (ie, IPV, help-seeking), which reflect multiple interlocking systems of oppression and privilege at the macrolevel (ie, racism, xenophobia, ableism, and classism).[17–19]

Abusive partners may use structural-level oppressive policies and practices as a way to control and cutoff survivors from resources. As an example, abusive partners may threaten to reveal a survivor's immigration status or refuse to sponsor permanent residency, thereby using xenophobic policies and practices against an IPV survivor.[17,20] Similarly, IPV survivors identifying as gender or sexual diverse may experience violence related to intersecting transphobia, genderism, and homophobia (eg, discrimination in health-care settings, partner threatening to "out" them),[21–23] which may be particularly harmful in the context of an increase in anti-lesbian, gay, bisexual, transgender, queer or questioning, intersex, asexual, and more (LGBTQIA) + laws occurring at the state level. Past studies has also shown that Black survivors are less likely to be believed and may not feel safe engaging law enforcement.[24,25] Survivors living in poverty are more likely to experience economic abuse and face housing insecurity[26] and experience abuse again after leaving a relationship.[27] Fundamentally, clinicians must work to disrupt the oppressive policies and practices that affect survivors' ability to access resources and thrive.

INTIMATE PARTNER VIOLENCE EXPOSURE INFLUENCES CHILD HEALTH

Decades of research have demonstrated that exposure to caregiver IPV influences child health, development, and thriving. Historically, articles have used a deficits-focused approach with long lists of negative child health outcomes; it is critical to shift to strengths-based approaches recognizing that IPV survivors do a remarkable job keeping their children safe and healthy. Further, children exposed to IPV are not "destined" to experience lifelong health impacts when they and their families are provided compassionate support and resources. With this framing in mind, IPV exposure has been associated with child mental health symptoms,[28] development delay,[29] chronic health concerns such as asthma,[30] and experiences of partner violence during adolescent relationships.[5] IPV is also associated with child abuse and neglect.[31,32] The impact of IPV on child and parent health further underscores the responsibility and opportunity for pediatric clinicians and systems in supporting IPV survivors.

HEALING-CENTERED ENGAGEMENT: A STRENGTHS-BASED FRAMEWORK

When considering how best to support parents and caregivers experiencing IPV, we recommend the use of a healing-centered engagement framework. Healing-centered engagement is a strength-based, antiracist framework that prioritizes healing, connection to social supports, and referrals to victim services agencies.[11,33–35] Core to healing-centered engagement is the recognition that trauma *and* healing occur at the individual and collective levels, and that trauma and healing may occur concurrently. Healing-centered engagement is strength-based—rather than asking survivors to relive their trauma, it focuses on highlighting their strengths and understanding their priorities. This may be particularly important when considering the intersectional experiences of IPV survivors from marginalized communities, who understandably may not trust health-care systems due to historical and current day discrimination and may not feel comfortable sharing IPV experiences in health-care spaces. A healing-centered approach can be used to both universally discuss IPV and support IPV survivors who share their experiences during a clinical visit, as detailed below.

UNIVERSAL EDUCATION AND RESOURCE PROVISION

Universal education and resource provision is an alternative to IPV screening, where *all* families are given brief education and resources around IPV rather than providing this information only to those who screen positive.[11,36,37] Such an approach shifts the paradigm away from disclosure-based strategies toward recognition that health-care settings must provide all families education and resources around this pervasive trauma. Providing resources to everyone also allows caregivers to share information with family and friends; even if they do not need resources, it is likely they will know someone experiencing IPV.

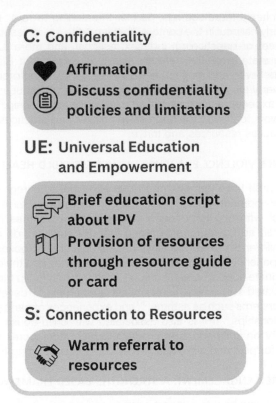

C: Confidentiality

♥ **Affirmation**

📋 **Discuss confidentiality policies and limitations**

UE: Universal Education and Empowerment

🗨 **Brief education script about IPV**

📖 **Provision of resources through resource guide or card**

S: Connection to Resources

🤝 **Warm referral to resources**

Fig. 1. CUES overview.

One universal education and resource provision framework is Confidentiality, University Education and Empowerment and Support (CUES)[36,37] whose steps are shown in **Fig. 1** and include discussing confidentiality, providing a brief script around IPV and resources to all families, and connecting families to more support if needed. CUES education scripts and resources can be IPV specific or part of a larger conversation about social and structural influences of health. Sample scripts are provided in an article by Ragavan and colleagues.[11] CUES approaches have been tested through cluster randomized clinical trials in other settings, including family planning clinics,[38] college health centers,[39] and school-based health centers.[40] These studies showed that the use of CUES is feasible and acceptable and increases self-efficacy to access resources, knowledge about IPV prevention, and, for adolescents, decreased violence victimization among those who reported IPV at baseline. Another similar universal education and resource provision approach is provide privacy, educate, ask, respect, and respond.[41] Passive materials such as handouts in bathrooms, posters on the walls, and easy access to helpline numbers can also be helpful to share information securely and privately around IPV.[42] Universal education and resource provision can be used in different pediatric health-care settings (eg, outpatient, inpatient, specialty, and emergency department) and during various types of health-care encounters. These approaches can also be used if the clinician has concern about IPV. Importantly, universal education and resource provision has not yet been tested in pediatric primary care clinics or with parent or caregiver IPV survivors, demonstrating an important area for future research.

Pediatric clinicians or settings may also choose a screening approach, where all caregivers are asked about IPV at regular intervals through written or face-to-face inquiry. Limited evidence exists for how best to implement parental and caregiver IPV screening in pediatric health-care settings although the United States Preventives Services Task Force does recommend screening for reproductive age women in adult settings.[43] If screening is used, we recommend it is included as part of universal education and resources and several challenges must be considered, particularly in the context of pediatric health-care settings.

- IPV survivors may not feel safe disclosing, due to concern about escalating abuse, child protective services (CPS) reporting, lack of trust in the health-care systems due to structural racism and historical trauma, among others.[44] As an example, in a study of more than 2000 IPV survivors, 35% said they did not ask for help because they were concerned their information would be reported to authority figures.[45] This concern is similarly reflected in recent data on screening in primary care settings more broadly, which showed only 8.5% of patients reported IPV and 65% of IPV screens resulted in patient refusal.[46]
- Screening tools often focus on physical, sexual, and psychological IPV and may not be inclusive toward survivors experiencing other types of controlling and abusive behaviors.
- Screening may add data around trauma to the electronic medical record, which may be unsafe particularly if the abusive partner is a coparent or caregiver and has access to patient portals.
- Face-to-face inquiry around IPV *must occur confidentially*, without verbal children (3 years or older) or other family members present.[47] Screening through telemedicine is not advised because privacy cannot be guaranteed.[11]
- Screening without support is not sufficient; if screening is preferred, resources must be available for survivors.

SUPPORTING INTIMATE PARTNER VIOLENCE SURVIVORS WHO DISCLOSE

In healing-centered engagement, disclosure is never the goal; however, when clinicians create healing spaces through universal education and resource provision, disclosures may happen. Disclosing IPV is a personal decision, and survivors may choose to disclose depending on their safety, supports, challenges, trust of the clinicians, and so forth. As described earlier, it is critical to remain survivor-centered; forcing a survivor to disclose may inadvertently perpetuate cycles of power and abuse.

Fig. 2 describes steps to support a survivor after they disclose (the "S" step in CUES). After a survivor shares their experiences, the clinician should provide validation and empathy and then should listen to the survivor, collaborating with them to share what feels most comfortable.[48] *Important for the pediatric setting is to never discuss IPV in front of other family members, including a verbal child.*[47] We recommend having another team member sit with the child or scheduling a follow-up call with the survivor at a time, which is safe for them. We also recommend providing connection to victim service agencies or other individuals with expertise in IPV.[49] Some survivors may prefer calling the victim service agency during the clinical visit and others may prefer to take the information and call when they feel ready. Clinicians can schedule follow-up appointments if this is helpful to the survivor and begin supporting IPV survivors with safety planning in health-care settings, if it is safe and feasible. Here, we offer words of caution particularly that safety planning and IPV experiences should never be discussed in front of other family members or friends, including verbal children. We highly recommended collaborating with a victim services

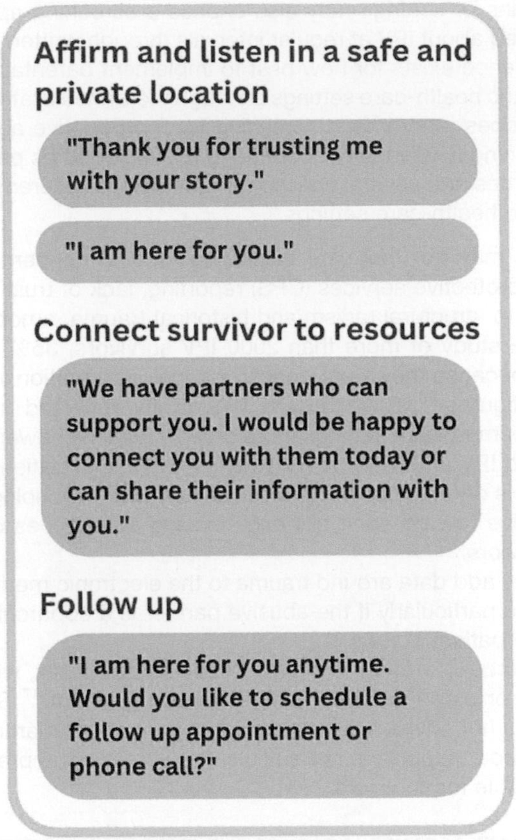

Affirm and listen in a safe and private location

"Thank you for trusting me with your story."

"I am here for you."

Connect survivor to resources

"We have partners who can support you. I would be happy to connect you with them today or can share their information with you."

Follow up

"I am here for you anytime. Would you like to schedule a follow up appointment or phone call?"

Fig. 2. Supporting a parent or caregiver who discloses IPV.

agency to provide safety planning, as described in subsequent sections. **Table 1** includes a safety-planning template.

Mandated Reporting to Child Protective Services

An important consideration in supporting IPV survivors in pediatric settings is mandated reporting to CPS. Clinicians must know their state laws because the majority of states do not require mandated reporting for children whose parents or caregivers are experiencing IPV, although some do, and laws are not static.[50] Interestingly, there is little best practice consensus around this topic. In a Delphi study of pediatric IPV experts (which did not include survivors themselves), consensus was reached that reporters should not file with exposure to IPV alone but should file with co-occurring child abuse and neglect.[51] There are multiple concerns around CPS reporting including escalation of abuse, further trauma for the family, and CPS reporting not leading to increased support or resources. In a survey on mandated reporting (including to CPS) of more than 2000 IPV survivors, 50% said a mandated report made their situation much worse.[45] It is also critically important for clinicians to understand how historical and current structural racism embedded within CPS and health-care systems has led to racial disproportionality within the CPS system, with children of color (particularly Black and Indigenous children) being overrepresented.[52,53] Clinicians should consider a transformative justice approach;

Table 1	
Resources for pediatric clinicians	
American Academy of Pediatrics Intimate Partner Violence website	https://www.aap.org/en/patient-care/intimate-partner-violence/
Futures Without Violence mandated reporting guidelines	https://promising.futureswithoutviolence.org/mandatory-reporting/
Futures Without Violence Issues Briefs	https://www.futureswithoutviolence.org/AAPIssueBriefs
Children's National Hospital Intimate Partner Violence training videos	https://www.aapdc.org/domestic-violence/
National Domestic Violence Hotline	https://www.thehotline.org/
Futures Without Violence guidelines for developing community-medical partnership	https://ipvhealthpartners.org/
Children's Hospital of Philadelphia video training	https://injury.research.chop.edu/blog/posts/new-resource-alert-addressing-domestic-violence-healthcare-settings
Healthy Children.org resource for parents	Stress and Violence at Home During Challenging Times—HealthyChildren.org

how can we prevent harm and violence without causing more harm and violence, and how do we hold the duality that we are mandated reporters but are reporting to (and from) systems rooted in racism, xenophobia, and other forms of oppression. Clinicians should review the work of Dorothy Roberts (and others; recent example is the book *Torn Apart*)[54] who share how to disrupt racial disproportionality within the CPS system and provide recommendations for grassroots, family-based, antiracist alternatives.

As we work to transform systems, we also recognize that clinicians may need to file CPS reports depending on state requirements and particularly in cases of co-occurring child abuse and neglect. In the Delphi study described above, consensus was reached around several best practices clinicians should consider when filing is indicated.[51]

- Survivors should be told why the report is needed.
- Survivors should be provided validation and affirmation that we are here to support them.
- Survivors be given the opportunity to file the report on their own (when possible, to allow them to control the situation).
- Clinicians should connect IPV survivors with resources and supports to develop safety plans.

Considered together, these recommendations underscore the importance of prioritizing supporting over simply reporting. Futures Without Violence has guidelines for pediatric clinicians about how best to support families in the context of mandated reporting (see **Table 1**).

Documentation of Intimate Partner Violence in the Electronic Medical Record

Documentation of parental or caregiver IPV in pediatric settings is unique because clinicians are documenting caregivers' experiences in the child's medical chart. Clinicians must be aware of potential implications of documentation, particularly in the context of the 21st Century Cures Act where patients have access to their and their children's medical records.[55,56] Documentation should be brief, objective, and whenever possible use coded languages (eg, family described stress).[57] Clinicians should not share documentation with information around IPV; in fact, IPV is one of the reasons where it is allowable to not share a note. It is our practice to document IPV in a separate, unshared noted rather than not sharing the full note. We also recommend carefully reviewing the full electronic medical record to ensure information around IPV is not inadvertently listed elsewhere (eg, problem list, social determinants of health screening, address, safe phone number, and so forth). Clinicians should always ask survivors how and where it is safe to document because they are the experts in their own safety and should be able to control how this information is documented in their child's medical chart.

COLLABORATION WITH VICTIM SERVICES AGENCIES
Victim Services Agencies

Victim services agencies support IPV survivors and are critical partners in the pediatric medical home and health-care infrastructure. Victim services agencies started as grassroots networks in the 1970s; now there are more than 1800 agencies serving 77,000 survivors daily.[58,59] Services exist at the national, state, and local levels. The national domestic violence hotline (https://www.thehotline.org/) has a 24/7 phone, text, and chat feature where survivors can connect with IPV advocates. Coalitions exist at the state level to provide coordination and collaboration among victim services providers. At the local level, most counties have at least one victim services agency, which offer a wide range of services as shown in **Fig. 3** (clinicians should check with their local agencies as services differ). Victim services agencies are staffed by IPV advocates, who are trained professionals specializing in confidential, healing-centered care and support survivors in various ways. As an example, they will often accompany survivors and their families to court hearings and medical visits. Pediatric clinicians should also be aware of culturally affirming agencies, defined as organizations centering the cultural experiences of their clients, which serve as important supports for IPV survivors with one or more marginalized identity.

Community-Medical Partnerships

Community-medical partnerships are bidirectional, reciprocal collaborations between victim services agencies and health-care settings and are integral to addressing IPV in health-care spaces. Community-medical partnerships facilitate survivor-centered care and response, warm handoffs to trusted partners, streamlined resource provision, and established procedures for care coordination across systems. Principles underlying the development of community-medical partnerships are synergistic with community-based participatory research approaches and include creating relationships rooted in transparency and trust, addressing individual and structural power

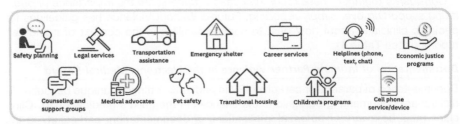

Fig. 3. Potential services available at victim services agencies.

inequities, promoting shared ownership and dissemination, and supporting mutual accountability and reciprocity.[17]

Guidelines for developing community-medical partnerships are described below. Please note that this is an iterative rather than linear process.

1. *Connect with a local IPV agency.* We recommend taking time to explore the agency's website, learning about the agency's history, services they provide, and upcoming events. After learning more, connect directly with the agency to meet and develop a blueprint for partnership development. Many agencies have a community outreach director or medical advocate that can assist with making these connections. Hosting bidirectional trainings with the IPV agency can facilitate partnership formation.

2. *Create an IPV workgroup.* Key to building community-medical partnerships is establishing an IPV work group. When developing this group, it is important to consider size, leadership, and membership, aligned with partnership principles. The optimal size for working groups can be tailored for the practice size; we recommend 4 to 15 with at least one champion who can support the group's growth. Team members should be multidisciplinary and include nurses, physicians, social workers, administrative personnel, and IPV advocates. Inclusion of IPV survivors is also critical but it is important to ensure that IPV survivors' voices are amplified and not silenced in the space by applying a power and privilege analysis to the group. We suggest that the group either be majority IPV survivors or have time set aside where IPV survivors can meet together with a skilled facilitator in their own space. When including IPV advocates and survivors, it is critical to compensate them for their time, expertise, and trauma as a baseline measure of reciprocity. This group will lead practice and policy decisions related to forming and sustaining the community-medical partnerships.

3. *Develop strategies to connect families to victim services agencies using survivor-centered approaches.* The IPV workgroup should develop processes for how to connect families to services, considering that survivors may wish to connect to resources in different ways. Some survivors may prefer calling an agency themselves; others may prefer calling the agency with the clinician in the room or having an advocate speak with them in real time. Warm referral systems—processes that directly connect the survivor to a point person at the victim services agency—should be developed. Warm handoffs build a relationship between the IPV survivor and advocate, which help with trust building, confidentiality, and safety.

4. *Consider creating a memorandum of understanding (MOU).* As this relationship is strengthened over time, explore models of partnership and consider creating an MOU to define the partnership. Futures Without Violence provides an exemplar MOU template (see **Table 1**), which can be revised to meet the partnership's specific needs.

5. *Consider colocated services.* As the community-medical partnership expands and grows, you may consider having colocated services, where IPV advocates work directly in clinical spaces. Examples of community-medical partnerships include the following:

   - Boston Children's Hospital offers on-call social workers through the AWAKE (Advocacy for Women and Kids Emergencies) program that provides free and confidential services for patients, their caregivers, and employees.[60]
   - Children's Mercy in Kansas City uses a multilevel approach to support IPV survivors that includes a hospital-based IPV advocacy program, a universal education/screening intervention, and staff education.[61]

- Children's Hospital of Philadelphia (CHOP) offers a multicomponent, collaborative program called STOP IPV with a local victim services agency. Full-time IPV specialists work on-site to offer direct services and provide trainings and system level support.[62]

TRAINING PEDIATRIC HEALTH-CARE PROVIDERS

Futures Without Violence, in collaboration with the American Academy of Pediatrics and UPMC Children's Hospital of Pittsburgh, published a recent brief prioritizing the need for clinician training to best support IPV survivors during and after the COVID-19 pandemic (see **Table 1**). Specifically, they recommend using a team-based approach that provides ongoing training to all clinicians, learners, and staff. In the subsequent sections, we review best practice recommendations for IPV training and strategies to incorporate IPV training into clinical practice.

Importance of Centering the Survivor's Voice

Core to this work is including IPV survivors because far too often "expert-developed" training does not include the voices of those with lived experience. Nicolaidis and colleagues demonstrated the impact of the *Voices of Survivors* documentary, along with a complementary workshop, which improved clinicians' knowledge, attitudes, empathy, and behaviors around IPV.[63] More recently, CHOP in collaboration with Temple University and Lutheran Settlement House, created a 4-part video series during which 3 IPV survivors detail their stories with IPV disclosure and provide advice to health-care providers (see **Table 1**). When centering survivor voices, it is critical to compensate them, amplify their strengths, and be inclusive to survivors with one or more marginalized identities.

Best Practices for Intimate Partner Violence Education in Clinical Settings

Despite recommendations around supporting IPV survivors in pediatric settings, there are limited data around IPV training content, delivery, or outcomes specific for pediatric settings. A scoping review of 56 published IPV curricula for medical trainees found that IPV was taught in medical school and residency; however, only 5 curricula were specific to pediatrics.[64] One example of a pediatric-based intervention for residents included education, screening prompts on patient medical forms, and hiring an on-site IPV counselor.[65] After implementation, pediatric residents demonstrate improved knowledge about IPV and how to access referral resources for survivors. In general, most curricula involved formal lectures and/or standardized patients. The most robust curriculum incorporated a didactic training during ethics class in first year, a small group session during a clinical rotation, and a small group session during students' outpatient clerkship. The review highlighted several commonly discussed topics including risk factors associated with IPV, screening and identification, physical examination concerns, barriers to disclosure, and legal protection and community resources. No study addressed universal education and/or the CUES intervention. Most studies reported subjective findings associated with provider attitudes, beliefs, and knowledge; few objectively measured clinical outcomes. The authors concluded that ideal IPV curriculum would use a multifaceted approach that includes didactic lectures, standardized patient encounters, cased-based approaches, and group reflection.

Intimate Partner Violence Educational Resources

Both Futures Without Violence and the AAP have several practical tools for supporting IPV survivors in pediatric health-care settings including sample scripts, patient

Table 2
MedEdPortal intimate partner violence training curricula

Title	Author/Date	Participants	Mode of Delivery	Type of Curriculum	Content of Curriculum
Talking to Patients About Sensitive Topics: Communication and Screening Techniques for Increasing the Reliability of Patient Self-Report	McBride,[68] 2012	First year medical students	Multi-modal small and large group sessions that cover 3 sensitive topics	90-min interactive didactic session followed by a 2-h clinical skills practice session using standardized patients	Addresses physician discomfort when discussing sensitive topics with patients by providing communication techniques that can decrease provider anxiety, improve reliability and accuracy of patient reports
Novice Health Care Students Learn Intimate Partner Violence Communication Skills through Standardized Patient Encounters	Jung et al.,[69] 2015	First-year and second-year medical students	Multimodal education as part of a 4-y longitudinal IPV curriculum	Year 1: 2 standardized patients during doctoring course Year 2: didactics, visit IPV shelter	IPV communication skills, mandatory reporting requirements, how to handle disclosure, and/or when a survivor is not ready for help
Health Education for Women and Children: A Community-Engaged Mutual Learning Curriculum for Health Trainees	Ragavan et al.,[70] 2016	IPV survivors residing at a translational housing program and health trainees	Large group workshops facilitated by health trainees (premedical students)	Ten 90-min workshops + 2 optional workshops, include didactics, group-based activities, and open discussion	Exercise, healthy cooking, parenting, managing stress, and so forth. Two optional workshops were on sexual coercion and health access

(continued on next page)

Table 2
(continued)

Title	Author/Date	Participants	Mode of Delivery	Type of Curriculum	Content of Curriculum
Addressing Interpersonal Violence as a Health Policy Question Using Interprofessional Community Educators	Clithero et al.,[71] 2016	Family medicine residents	Small and large group session led by community interprofessional educator at a local family advocacy center	2-h case review	Examines a clinical encounter with a patient experiencing IPV and homelessness and the implications of existing policy on the delivery of health-care services
Intimate Partner Violence Screening and Counseling: An Introductory Session for Health Care Professionals	Schrier et al., 2017	Medical students	Flipped classroom model. Small groups of 8 students paired with one physician and on social-behavioral science faculty member	Prereading material, 3-h clinical skills course including role-plays and open discussion. Standardized patient 1-y posteducation	IPV screening and counseling using a checklist companion for tips on how to navigate the conversation, using a motivational interviewing framework
A Novel Intimate Partner Violence Curriculum for Internal Medicine Residents: Development, Implementation, and Evaluation	Insetta et al.,[72] 2020	First-year internal medicine residents	Small and large group sessions in classroom setting led by several interprofessional educators	Part 1 (60 min): TEDtalk or in-person discussion with social worker from IPV shelter, didactics, and case review. Part 2 (90 min): didactics, role-play	Part 1 focused on foundational information about IPV such as the prevalence, red flags, health consequences, recommendations for documenting, reporting, and access to local services. Part 2 focused on how to apply this information in clinical settings

---

Box 1
Recommendations for creating healing-centered systems

Prioritize development of comprehensive services and supports for IPV survivors (rather than just screening)

Develop and sustain funded programs to colocate IPV advocates in pediatric health-care settings to more easily facilitate warm handoffs

Partner with IPV survivors and advocates when developing service recommendations

Invest in community-medical partnerships and compensate victim services agencies who support patients

Provide survivor-centered training to all clinicians and staff

Develop systems for clinicians to privately speak with IPV survivors in pediatric health-care settings, without further traumatizing the child(ren). One potential option is a greater investment in child life specialists who can support children while the clinician is speaking with the parent or caregiver

Reimburse follow-up phone calls with IPV survivors so clinicians can further support them

Invest in healing for clinicians themselves, to address moral injury and vicarious trauma

Continue to interrogate institutional policies and practices to ensure they are strength-based, healing-centered, and rooted in principles of disrupting structural oppressions and making transformational change

---

vignettes, videos, and expert perspectives. Children's National Medical Center has developed online modules for pediatric clinicians that reviews specific cases of IPV, describes how best to respond to such cases, and identifies resources available to survivors in these situations (see **Table 1**). MedEdPortal, an open-access journal published by the Association of American Medical Colleges has several peer-reviewed IPV educational curricula available that one can implement within their pediatric clinical setting (synthesized in **Table 2**).

Creating Healing-Centered Systems

Much of what is offered above focuses on healing-centered providers or clinics, which are critically needed. However, to be truly transformative health-care systems also need to become more healing-centered and prioritize funding and resources toward supporting IPV survivors and their children.[66] There is a current priority being placed on systems-wide social determinants of health screening (which may include IPV) due to regulations from the Joint Commission, Centers for Medicare and Medicaid, and US News and World Reports.[66] This work has focused on screening, although more comprehensive systems-based programs to address SDOH are needed.[67] Leveraging this momentum, we now delineate several recommendations for health-care systems in Text **Box 1**. Although not an exhaustive list, these recommendations demonstrate the need to invest money, time, and resources in IPV prevention rather than shifting the burden onto individual providers.

SUMMARY AND KEY TAKE HOME POINTS FOR PEDIATRIC CLINICIANS

Pediatric clinicians and health-care settings have an urgent responsibility to support IPV survivors and their children. Key take home points are listed below.

1. IPV is pervasive and rooted in multilevel power and control, including through partners using structural-level oppressive policies and practices.

2. As an alternative to screening, we recommend the use of universal education and resource provision, with additional supports provided if a parent or caregiver discloses experiencing IPV.
3. Developing community-medical partnerships with victim services agencies can offer real-time support for IPV survivors.
4. Comprehensive, mandatory, yearly, strength-based, multidisciplinary, and inclusive training around IPV for pediatric trainees, clinicians, and staff is needed to ensure provision of healing-centered care within pediatric health-care settings.
5. Use of healing-centered approaches both as a framework for clinician–patient communication and to reimagine health systems more broadly is critical to amplify survivor strengths and support families.

ACKNOWLEDGMENTS

The authors would like to thank Erin Mickievicz, BA for her assistance in creating the figures for this article.

FUNDING

Dr Ragavan is supported by a K23 from the National Institute on Child Health and Human Development (K23HD104925).

DISCLOSURE

Drs M.I. Ragavan and A. Murray have no conflicts of interest to disclose.

REFERENCES

1. Leemis RW, Friar N, Khatiwada S, Chen MS, Kresnow M, Smith SG, Caslin S, & Basile KC. The National Intimate Partner and Sexual Violence Survey: 2016/2017 Report on Intimate Partner Violence. Atlanta, GA: National Center for Injury Prevention and Control, Centers for Disease Control and Prevention; 2022. Retrieved from: The National Intimate Partner and Sexual Violence Survey: 2016/2017 Report on Intimate Partner Violence (cdc.gov).
2. Garthe RC, Kaur A, Rieger A, et al. Dating violence and peer victimization among male, female, transgender, and gender-expansive youth. Pediatrics 2021;147(4). e2020004317.
3. Dank M, Lachman P, Zweig JM, et al. Dating violence experiences of lesbian, gay, bisexual, and transgender youth. J Youth Adolesc 2014;43(5):846–57.
4. Hamby S, Finkelhor D, Turner H, et al. Children's exposure to intimate partner violence and other family violence. US Department of Justice; 2010.
5. Ragavan MI, Culyba AJ, Shaw D, et al. Social support, exposure to parental intimate partner violence, and relationship abuse among marginalized youth. J Adolesc Health 2020;67(1):127–30.
6. Randell KA, Ragavan MI. Intimate partner violence: identification and response in pediatric health care settings. Clin Pediatr (Phila) 2020;59(2):109–15.
7. Thackeray JD, Hibbard R, Dowd MD. Committee on child abuse and neglect; committee on injury, violence, and poison prevention. intimate partner violence: the role of the pediatrician. Pediatrics 2010;125(5):1094–100.
8. Domestic Abuse Intervention Program. Understanding the Power and Control Wheel. Available at: https://www.theduluthmodel.org/wheels/. Accessed November 18, 2019.

9. Stylianou AM. Economic abuse within intimate partner violence: a review of the literature. Violence Vict 2018;33(1):3–22.

10. Miller SL, Smolter NL. "Paper abuse": when all else fails, batterers use procedural stalking. Violence Against Women 2011;17(5):637–50.

11. Ragavan MI, Garcia R, Berger RP, et al. Supporting intimate partner violence survivors and their children during the COVID-19 pandemic. Pediatrics 2020;146(3): e20201276.

12. Ragavan MI, Risser L, Duplessis V, et al. The impact of the COVID-19 pandemic on the needs and lived experiences of intimate partner violence survivors in the united states: advocate perspectives. Violence Against Women 2022;28(12–13): 3114–34.

13. Wyckoff KG, Narasimhan S, Stephenson K, et al. "COVID gave him an opportunity to tighten the reins around my throat": perceptions of COVID-19 movement restrictions among survivors of intimate partner violence. BMC Publ Health 2023; 23(1):199.

14. Beeble ML, Bybee D, Sullivan CM. Abusive men's use of children to control their partners and ex-partners. Eur Psychol 2007;12(1).

15. Risser L, Berger RP, Renov V, et al. Supporting children experiencing family violence during the COVID-19 pandemic: IPV and CPS provider perspectives. Acad Pediatr 2022;22(5):842–9.

16. Ragavan MI, Query LA, Bair-Merritt M, et al. Expert perspectives on intimate partner violence power and control in pediatric healthcare settings. Acad Pediatr 2021;21(3):548–56.

17. Ragavan MI, Thomas KA, Fulambarker A, et al. Exploring the needs and lived experiences of racial and ethnic minority domestic violence survivors through community-based participatory research: a systematic review. Trauma Violence Abuse 2020;21(5):946–63.

18. Crenshaw K. Mapping the margins: intersectionality, identity politics, and violence against women of color. Stanford Law Rev 1991;43:1241–99, 29.

19. Sokoloff NJ, Dupont I. Domestic violence at the intersections of race, class, and gender: challenges and contributions to understanding violence against marginalized women in diverse communities. Violence Against Women 2005;11(1): 38–64.

20. Hulley J, Bailey L, Kirkman G, et al. Intimate partner violence and barriers to help-seeking among black, asian, minority ethnic and immigrant women: a qualitative metasynthesis of global research [published online ahead of print, 2022 Feb 2]. Trauma Violence Abuse 2022. https://doi.org/10.1177/15248380211050590. 15248380211050590.

21. Rogers M. Breaking down barriers: exploring the potential for social care practice with trans survivors of domestic abuse. Health Soc Care Community 2016;24(1): 68–76.

22. Kattari SK, Kattari L, Lacombe-Duncan A, et al. Differential experiences of sexual, physical, and emotional intimate partner violence among transgender and gender diverse adults. J Interpers Violence 2022;37(23–24):NP23281–305.

23. Gamarel KE, Jadwin-Cakmak L, King WM, et al. Stigma experienced by transgender women of color in their dating and romantic relationships: implications for gender-based violence prevention programs. J Interpers Violence 2022; 37(9–10):NP8161–89.

24. Monterrosa AE. How race and gender stereotypes influence help-seeking for intimate partner violence. J Interpers Violence 2021;36(17–18):NP9153–74.

25. Decker MR, Holliday CN, Hameeduddin Z, et al. "You do not think of me as a human being": Race and gender inequities intersect to discourage police reporting of violence against women. J Urban Health 2019;96(5):772–83.

26. Goodman LA, Smyth KF, Borges AM, et al. When crises collide: how intimate partner violence and poverty intersect to shape women's mental health and coping? Trauma Violence Abuse 2009;10(4):306–29.

27. Bybee D, Sullivan CM. Predicting re-victimization of battered women 3 years after exiting a shelter program. Am J Community Psychol 2005;36(1–2):85–96.

28. Holt S, Buckley H, Whelan S. The impact of exposure to domestic violence on children and young people: a review of the literature. Child Abuse Negl 2008; 32(8):797–810.

29. Neamah HH, Sudfeld C, McCoy DC, et al. Intimate partner violence, depression, and child growth and development. Pediatrics 2018;142(1):e20173457.

30. Wang E, Zahid S, Moudgal AN, et al. Intimate partner violence and asthma in pediatric and adult populations. Ann Allergy Asthma Immunol 2022;128(4):361–78.

31. Hamby S, Finkelhor D, Turner H, et al. The overlap of witnessing partner violence with child maltreatment and other victimizations in a nationally representative survey of youth. Child Abuse Negl 2010;34(10):734–41.

32. Tullberg E, Vaughon W. Revisiting the co-occurrence of intimate partner violence and child maltreatment. J Interpers Violence 2023;38(3–4):2957–82.

33. Miller E. Healing-centered engagement: fostering connections rather than forcing disclosures. In: Ginsburgy KR, Brett Z, McClain R, editors. Reaching Teens: strength-based, trauma-Sensitive, Resilience-building communication strategies rooted in positive youth development. Elk Grove Village, IL: American Academy of Pediatrics; 2020.

34. Ginwright S. The future of healing: Shifting from trauma informed care to healing centered engagement. 2018; https://ginwright.medium.com/the-future-of-healing-shifting-from-trauma-informed-care-to-healing-centered-engagement-634f557ce 69c. Accessed date 21 May 2021.

35. Ragavan MI, Miller E. Healing-Centered Care for Intimate Partner Violence Survivors and Their Children. Pediatrics 2022;149(6).

36. Miller E, McCaw B. Intimate Partner Violence. N Engl J Med 2019;380(9):850–7.

37. Futures Without Violence. CUES: Addressing domestic and sexual violence in health settings Retrieved from: CUES.pdf (futureswithoutviolence.org). Accessed date 3 March 2023.

38. Miller E, McCauley HL, Decker MR, et al. Implementation of a family planning clinic-based partner violence and reproductive coercion intervention: provider and patient perspectives. Perspect Sex Reprod Health 2017;49(2):85–93.

39. Miller E, Jones KA, McCauley HL, et al. Cluster randomized trial of a college health center sexual violence intervention. Am J Prev Med 2020;59(1):98–108.

40. Miller E, Goldstein S, McCauley HL, et al. A school health center intervention for abusive adolescent relationships: a cluster RCT. Pediatrics 2015;135(1):76–85.

41. CommonSpirit Health, HEAL Trafficking, Pacific Survivor Center. PEARR Tool: Trauma-Informed Approach to Victim Assistance in Health Care Settings. 2020. Available at: PEARR-Tool-2020.pdf (healtrafficking.org). Last Accessed June 2, 2021.

42. Randell KA, Sherman A, Walsh I, et al. Intimate partner violence educational materials in the acute care setting: acceptability and impact on female caregiver attitudes toward screening. Pediatr Emerg Care 2021;37(1):e37–41.

43. US Preventive Services Task Force, Curry SJ, Krist AH, Owens DK, et al. Screening for intimate partner violence, elder abuse, and abuse of vulnerable

adults: US preventive services task force final recommendation statement. JAMA 2018;320(16):1678–87.

44. Othman S, Goddard C, Piterman L. Victims' barriers to discussing domestic violence in clinical consultations: a qualitative enquiry. J Interpers Violence 2014;29(8): 1497–513.

45. Lippy C, Jumarali SN, Nnawulezi NA, et al. The impact of mandatory reporting laws on survivors of intimate partner violence: intersectionality, help-seeking and the need for change. J Fam Violence 2019;35:255–67.

46. Perone HR, Dietz NA, Belkowitz J, et al. Intimate partner violence: analysis of current screening practices in the primary care setting. Fam Pract 2022;39(1):6–11.

47. Zink T, Levin L, Wollan P, et al. Mothers' comfort with screening questions about sensitive issues, including domestic violence. J Am Board Fam Med 2006;19(4): 358–67.

48. Chang JC, Decker MR, Moracco KE, et al. Asking about intimate partner violence: advice from female survivors to health care providers. Patient Educ Counsel 2005;59(2):141–7.

49. Dichter ME, Ogden SN, Tuepker A, et al. Survivors' input on health care-connected services for intimate partner violence. J Womens Health (Larchmt) 2021;30(12):1744–50.

50. Mandatory reporters of child abuse and neglect. Washington, DC: U.S. Department of Health and Human Services, Children's Bureau; 2019.

51. Ragavan MI, Skinner CM, Killough EF, et al. Child protective services reports in the context of intimate partner violence: a delphi process examining best practices. Acad Pediatr 2022;22(5):833–41.

52. Cenat JM, McIntee S-E, Mukunzi JN, et al. Overrepresentation of Black children in the child welfare system: a systematic review to understand and better act. Child Youth Serv Rev 2021;120:105714.

53. Cross TL. Racial disproportionality and disparities among American Indian and Alaska Native populations. In: Dettlaff, editor. Racial disproportionality and Disparities in the child Welfare system. Cham: Springer International Publishing; 2021. p. 99–124.

54. Roberts D. Torn Apart: how the child Welfare system Destroys Black families and how Abolition can build a safer World. New York, NY: Basic Books; 2022.

55. Congress.gov. HR 34—21st Century Cures Act. Accessed on 3/3/2023. Available at: https://www.congress.gov/bill/114th-congress/house-bill/34/.

56. Shum M, Asnes AG, Jubanyik K, et al. The 21st century cures act: affecting the safety of intimate partner violence survivors and their children. Ann Emerg Med 2022;79(5):503–4.

57. Randell KA, Ragavan MI, Query LA, et al. Intimate partner violence and the pediatric electronic health record: a qualitative study. Acad Pediatr 2022;22(5): 824–32.

58. Macy RJ, Giattina M, Sangster TH, et al. Domestic violence and sexual assault services: Inside the black box. Aggress Violent Behav 2009;14(5):359–73.

59. National Network to End Domestic Violence (NNEDV). (2020, March 10). 14th Annual Domestic Violence Counts Report. Retrieved March 17, 2021, Available at: https://nnedv.org/wp-content/uploads/2020/03/Library_Census-2019_Report_web.pdf. Accessed July 1, 2021.

60. Rahman R, Huysman C, Ross AM, et al. Intimate partner violence and the COVID-19 pandemic. Pediatrics 2022;149(6). e2021055792.

61. CHILDREN'S MERCY NEED TO ADD.

62. Children's Hospital of Philadelphia. Center for Violence Prevention. Available at: https://violence.chop.edu/research-and-programs/intimate-partner-violence-prevention. Accessed date 03 March 2023.
63. Nicolaidis C, Curry M, Gerrity M. Measuring the impact of the Voices of Survivors program on health care workers' attitudes toward survivors of intimate partner violence. J Gen Intern Med 2005;20(8):731–7.
64. Ghaith S, Voleti SS, Ginsberg Z, et al. A scoping review of published intimate partner violence curricula for medical trainees. J Womens Health (Larchmt) 2022;31(11):1596–613.
65. McColgan MD, Cruz M, McKee J, et al. Results of a multifaceted Intimate Partner Violence training program for pediatric residents. Child Abuse Negl 2010;34(4): 275–83.
66. Toccalino D, Haag HL, Estrella MJ, et al. The intersection of intimate partner violence and traumatic brain injury: findings from an emergency summit addressing system-level changes to better support women survivors. J Head Trauma Rehabil 2022;37(1):E20–9.
67. Ragavan MI, Garg A, Raphael JL. Creating healing-centered health systems by reimagining social needs screening and supports. JAMA Pediatr 2023;77(6): 555–6.
68. McBride R. Talking to patients about sensitive topics: Communication and screening techniques for increasing the reability of patient self-report. MedEdPortal 2012. https://doi.org/10.15766/mep_2374-8265.9089.
69. Jung D, Kavanagh M, Joyce B, et al. Novice health care students learn intimate partner violence communication skills through standardized patient encounters. MedEdPortal 2015. https://doi.org/10.15766/mep_2374-8265.9977.
70. Ragavan M, Karpel H, Bogetz A, et al. Health Education for Women and Children: A Community-Engaged Mutual Learning Curriculum for Health Trainees. MedEdPORTAL 2016;12:10492. https://doi.org/10.15766/mep_2374-8265.10492.
71. Clithero A, Albright D, Bissell E, et al. Addressing Interpersonal Violence as a Health Policy Question Using Interprofessional Community Educators. MedEdPORTAL 2016;12:10516. https://doi.org/10.15766/mep_2374-8265.10516.
72. Insetta ER, Christmas C. A Novel Intimate Partner Violence Curriculum for Internal Medicine Residents: Development, Implementation, and Evaluation. MedEdPORTAL 2020;16:10905. https://doi.org/10.15766/mep_2374-8265.10905.

The Health Care Provider's Role in Addressing Adolescent Relationship Abuse

Lenore Jarvis, MD, MEd[a], Kimberly A. Randell, MD, MSc[b,c,d],*

KEYWORDS

- Adolescent relationship abuse • Teen dating violence • Reproductive coercion
- Violence prevention • Healing-centered engagement • Power • Control

KEY POINTS

- Adolescent relationship abuse (ARA) is highly prevalent and may include sexual, psychological, and cyber abuse, and reproductive coercion.
- ARA, as well as other trauma and stressors, should be considered when adolescents have mental health concerns, school difficulties, somatic complaints, substance abuse, sexually transmitted infections, or pregnancy.
- Health care providers have opportunity for ARA prevention using a universal education approach that provides information on healthy and unhealthy relationship behaviors and ARA resources.
- Adolescents should be made aware of any limits to patient-provider confidentiality and provided opportunity for resource connection that is not disclosure dependent.
- A shared decision-making approach when responding to ARA disclosure may facilitate patient-provider trust, safety, resource utilization, and adolescent autonomy.

INTRODUCTION

Adolescent relationship abuse (ARA; also called "teen dating violence") is a significant public health concern that affects millions of adolescents in the United States and globally.[1–3] ARA is characterized by a pattern of behavior in which a person abuses their partner within a dating relationship wherein one or both partners is a minor; it may include one or more types of abusive behavior, such as physical, sexual, psychological, or cyber abuse and reproductive coercion (**Table 1**).[4] Cyber ARA refers to the use of technology to harass and control a dating partner; importantly, a partner does not need to be physically present to use these behaviors.[5] Reproductive coercion is

[a] Children's National Hospital, The George Washington University School of Medicine and Health Sciences, 111 Michigan Avenue Northwest, Washington, DC 20010, USA; [b] Children's Mercy Kansas City, 2401 Gillham Road, Kansas City, MO 64110, USA; [c] University of Missouri-Kansas City School of Medicine, Kansas City, MO, USA; [d] University of Kansas School of Medicine, Kansas City, KS, USA
* Corresponding author.
E-mail address: karandell@cmh.edu

Pediatr Clin N Am 70 (2023) 1087–1102
https://doi.org/10.1016/j.pcl.2023.06.006
0031-3955/23/© 2023 Elsevier Inc. All rights reserved.

Table 1
Examples of abusive relationship behaviors[4,62]

Anger/Emotional Abuse	• Puts partner down • Makes partner feel badly about themselves • Name calling • Humiliates partner in front of their friends • Makes partner think they are crazy • Makes partner feel guilty • Extreme jealousy • Gets angry quickly and violently
Isolation/Exclusion	• Pressures partner to choose between them and friends/family • Controls what partner does or who they see/talk to • Limiting outside involvement • Using jealousy to justify actions
Violates Privacy	• Reads partner's texts and social networking sites • Goes through partner's belongings (eg, purse, locker, backpack) without permission • Forced sharing of passwords • Harassment via social media platforms • Stalking via GPS technology
Limits Independence	• Controls what partner wears • Makes all the decisions in the relationship
Threats and Intimidation	• Intimidation via looks, actions, gestures, or property destruction • Abuses pets • Displays weapons • Threatens to harm partner and/or their friends/family • Threatens to report partner or their family to immigration services • Threatens to "out" partner's sexual orientation or gender identity • Threatens suicide if the partner leaves the relationship
Minimizes/Denies/Blames	• Makes light of the abuse, not taking the concerns seriously • Says the abuse did not happen • Shifts blame for the abusive behavior • Apologizes
Using Social Status/ Peer Pressure	• Tells partner they are lucky to have them • Tells partner they are nobody without them • Threatens to spread rumors about partner • Emphasizes or defines gender roles in the relationship, including asserting male privilege
Sexual Coercion	• Manipulation or threats to get sex • Getting partner drunk or drugged to have sex • Transactional sex (exchange of sexual acts for housing, drugs, financial support, or other material good)
Reproductive Coercion	• Interference with access to birth control • Threats or force to coerce pregnancy or pregnancy outcome • Condom refusal or sabotage

the exertion of power and control over a partner's reproductive choices, such as coerced pregnancy or control over outcomes of a pregnancy.[4] Reproductive coercion may include interference with contraceptive methods or psychological or physical coercion to have unprotected sex. Additionally, emerging work suggests that ARA may also be characterized by transactional sex (ie, exchange of sexual acts for money, housing, food, or other goods) or economic abuse.[6–8] The underlying commonality among these abusive behaviors is the exertion of power and control by one partner over another.[9]

ARA affects adolescents regardless of gender, race, ethnicity, sexual orientation, or socioeconomic status.[1,2] Among US high school students reporting dating, approximately 1 in 12e report past-year physical ARA; 1 in 12 report past-year sexual ARA.[1] Sixty nine percent of adolescents who have dated in the past year reported lifetime ARA victimization; 63% reported lifetime perpetration.[10] Female adolescents aged 15 years and older are at the highest risk, compared to younger adolescents.[10] Although victimization and perpetration are common among both male and female youth, females are more likely to experience sexual abuse and more severe physical abuse.[1] Some adolescent males may have gender-typed beliefs that increase risk for ARA perpetration through an emphasis on male power and men as tough, aggressive, emotionally disengaged, and having sexual prerogative in romantic relationships; this may lead to increased risk for perpetrating ARA as a means of enacting power in their relationships.[11] Reproductive coercion has been reported by 1 in 5 high school females.[12] Prevalence of reported cyber ARA varies widely, depending on assessment methodology.[5]

Although ARA occurs within all demographic groups, adolescents belonging to structurally marginalized groups may be at higher risk for ARA victimization. Current studies suggest that lesbian, gay, and bisexual adolescents were significantly more likely (35% vs 8%) than their heterosexual counterparts to experience ARA.[13] Transgender adolescents have also reported higher rates of ARA victimization, compared to cisgender peers.[1,13] Such disparities should be recognized as resulting from systemic and structural marginalization (eg, homophobia, transphobia) rather than characteristics of a specific group that make these adolescents more likely to be victimized.[14] Recent evidence suggests adolescents from minoritized racial and ethnic groups are not more likely to experience ARA than their White peers.[1,10]

Providers who care for adolescents must be prepared to promote healthy relationships and support ARA survivors given that adolescents experiencing ARA are at increased risk for negative health and psychosocial outcomes. These include sexually transmitted infections (STIs), unplanned or unwanted pregnancy, depression, suicidality, and school dropout (**Box 1**).[15–19] Further, adolescents experiencing ARA are more likely to engage in risk behaviors including peer violence, sexual risk behaviors, and substance use.[17,19,20] Among adolescent homicides in 2003 to 2016, 7% were intimate partner homicide, among which 90% of the victims were female.[21] Among US adults reporting physical or sexual intimate partner violence (IPV) or stalking by an intimate partner, 27% of the females and 21% of the males first experienced partner violence before the age of 18 years.[2]

DISCUSSION
General Considerations

It is important to consider several concepts that apply broadly across work with adolescents: adolescent development, healing-centered engagement, intersectionality, co-occurring forms of violence, and ARA prevention.

Adolescent development
Adolescence is a critical developmental period with significant physical, intellectual, social, and emotional development and growth. During this period, adolescents transition from perceiving the world in immediate, concrete terms, gaining capacity for increasingly abstract thought. Cognitive brain development progresses throughout adolescence, enabling adolescents to better understand and solve complex problems,

---

Box 1
Indicators of possible ARA

Isolation from former friends and/or little social contact with anyone but the dating partner

Unexplained bruises or injuries

Sexually transmitted infection

Pregnancy

Somatic complaints (eg, headache, abdominal pain)

Noticeable change in weight, demeanor, or physical appearance

Depression

Disordered eating

Suicidality

Sudden request for school schedule change

Poor school attendance

Poor academic performance and/or new disciplinary problems at school

School dropout

Substance use

Physical fights with peers

Sexual risk behaviors

Lack of interest in former extracurricular activities

Excessive texting, calling, sexting

---

have improved judgement, and plan for the future.[22] This brain development is shaped by a host of factors, including genetics, hormones, nutrition, sleep, the environment and community, childhood experiences, relationships, substance use and abuse, and trauma.[23] Adolescents may have a stronger emotional response to situations and images that are emotionally loaded. Although adolescence is a time of risk and increased vulnerability to violence, this capacity for risk-taking is essential for adolescents to accomplish the transition adulthood.[24] This transition encompasses testing and asserting independence from parents and increasing importance of peer relationships, including exploration of romantic relationships.

Healing-centered engagement

Healing-centered engagement is a holistic, trauma-informed, positive youth development approach that is broadly applicable to adolescent health care.[25,26] Healing-centered engagement emphasizes both trauma and resilience as universal experiences, recognizes that trauma and healing occur within relationships, and empowers adolescents to actively participate in their healing process. This approach emphasizes the strengths of both the individual adolescent and their community and highlights the role of relationships, culture, spirituality, and civic action in individual and collective healing. The ARA-specific recommendations that follow are made from the context of healing-centered engagement and prioritize relationships, connection to resources, empowerment, and autonomy. General practices that may facilitate healing-centered engagement in health care settings include ensuring awareness of limits to patient-provider confidentiality, opportunity for resource connection that is not disclosure dependent, and a shared decision-making approach when ARA is disclosed. These practices can foster patient-provider trust, empower adolescents, and minimize risk for potential unintended harm related to health care provision.

Intersectionality

Health care providers must consider the intersectional impacts of overlapping identities, particularly those aspects of identity that are structurally marginalized.[27] Multiple influences on behavior occur across individual, relationship, community, and societal levels.[28] Experiences of ARA and related resource use are influenced by structural oppression related to racism, homophobia, xenophobia, ableism, and sexism. Adolescents within marginalized communities are impacted by both their personal experiences of discrimination as well as the intergenerational repercussions of historical trauma. They may experience unique forms of power and control or additional barriers to help-seeking. For example, lesbian, gay, bisexual, transgender, and questioning (or queer) (LGBTQ) + adolescents experiences of ARA and help-seeking may be impacted by fear regarding public knowledge of their gender and/or sexuality.[29] Black and Latinx adolescents may be less likely to utilize formal victim services, such as police, compared to informal resources such as family and friends.[30] For adolescents from immigrant communities, ARA and help-seeking may be impacted by language, culture, and immigration status.[31]

Co-occurring forms of violence

Different forms of interpersonal violence, including adolescent violence, child abuse and neglect, IPV, and sexual violence are strongly connected.[32] Individuals who are victims of one form of violence are likely to experience other forms of violence, all of which may impact both individuals and communities across generations.[33] Different forms of violence share common risk factors, protective factors, and consequences, including negative health outcomes.[32] Therefore, focusing on ARA prevention may have cross-cutting effects.

Adolescent relationship abuse prevention

Health care providers have opportunities to address ARA along the full spectrum of prevention, including primary, secondary, and tertiary prevention.[34] Primary prevention focuses on supporting healthy relationship behaviors and avoidance of ARA entirely. Such efforts include education about healthy relationship behaviors and addressing gender norms while simultaneously reducing environmental risks and increasing protective environment and resilience factors. Secondary prevention focuses on minimizing the impact of ARA through early identification and immediate resource provision. Tertiary prevention seeks to mitigate the long-term effects of ARA.

Supporting Healthy Adolescent Relationships in Health Care Settings

Health care settings may provide unique opportunities for ARA prevention. However, evidence suggests that providers frequently miss such opportunities; adolescents, their parents, and primary care providers report that health care providers uncommonly discuss healthy relationship behaviors or ARA with adolescents.[35] Providers may use varied strategies for ARA prevention depending on the presence or absence of ARA indicators, adolescent disclosure, and type of abuse disclosed. Recommendations described in detail are summarized in **Box 2**. Resources to support implementation of these recommendations are provided in **Boxes 3** and **4**.

Universal education

A universal education approach that reinforces healthy and unhealthy relationship behaviors as well as information on ARA resources enables ARA prevention at any health

---

Box 2
Clinical care pearls

- A universal education approach, in which all adolescents are provided with resources to support healthy relationships and address ARA, enables health care providers to support adolescents experiencing ARA even in the absence of disclosure.

- Providers should consider ARA, as well as other trauma and stressors, when they identify substance abuse, mental health concerns, somatic complaints, or difficulties in school.

- Providers should inform adolescents of limits to confidentiality, including mandatory reporting requirements, before discussing ARA.

- Assure a safe space and privacy in both conversation and clinical examination.

- When examining an adolescent ask for consent, explain what will be done, how it will be done, and why; provide choices, allow the patient to decline, and observe body language carefully.

- Robust response to ARA disclosure should include validation and resource provision, including point-of-care harm reduction resources such as STI testing/treatment, pregnancy testing, and emergency contraception and a warm hand-off to victim services.

- Internet-based and text-based services offer opportunities for resource connection even in resource-poor health care settings.

- Shared decision-making that engages adolescents around notification of trusted adults and mandated reporting after ARA disclosure facilitates patient-provider trust, supports adolescent autonomy, and can help ensure adolescent safety.

- Supporting parents to engage in conversations and limit-settings around dating relationships is a key component of ARA prevention.

---

care visit. This approach recognizes that adolescents may not feel comfortable or safe disclosing ARA due to confidentiality concerns; isolation, shame, or embarrassment; fear of partner's retaliation or a parent's disapproval; and lack of trust in professionals.[30,31,36] Thus, universal education empowers adolescents to access resources at the time that is right for them by facilitating connection to ARA resources that is not disclosure driven. Additionally, universal education may equip adolescents to provide more robust support to peers who experience abuse. Given that adolescents often talk to their friends before or rather than speaking to adults, they may serve as an important resource and support for their peers.[36]

Evidence suggests that universal education using a Confidentiality-Universal education-Empowerment-Support (CUES) approach is effective. The healthcare education assessment and response for teen relationships (HEART) intervention uses a CUES approach for universal ARA education in school health centers.[4] Adolescents at school health centers that implemented HEART were more likely to recognize sexually coercive behaviors, disclose ARA, and, among those reporting ARA at baseline, less likely to report ARA at follow-up.[37] Additional studies showed the CUES approach is also effective in family planning clinics.[38,39] **Box 4** provides a suggested universal education script; the HEART pocket safety card is available for download from Futures Without Violence.[40] Providers may also choose to use a locally developed list of resources that includes local and national resources for ARA and other adolescent concerns.

Universal screening
Although the United States Preventive Services Task Force recommends screening women of reproductive age for IPV and referral of survivors to support services,[41]

Box 3
ARA resources

Local Resources
- State Coalitions: https://ncadv.org/state-coalitions

National Resources for Adolescents and Adult Allies
  ARA:
  - National Dating Abuse Helpline: 1-866-331-9474, chat online at loveisrespect.org, or text "loveis" to 22522.
  - General ARA and healthy relationship information:
      www.thatsnotcool.com
      Break The Cycle: www.breakthecycle.org
  - Cyber abuse: www.athinline.org
  Sexual Assault:
  - National Sexual Assault Hotline: 1-800-6564673, www.rainn.org
  Suicide:
  - National Suicide Prevention Lifeline: 1-800-273-8255 (TALK), www.suicidepreventionlifeline.org
  LGBTQ+:
  - The Trevor Project – Crisis & Suicide Prevention Lifeline for LGBTQ+ Youth: www.thetrevorproject.org, 1-866-488-7386
  - It Gets Better Project: www.itgetsbetter.org
  - Trans Lifeline: www.translifeline.org
  Adolescent Reproductive and Sexual Health (including contraception options):
  - Bedsider: www.bedsider.org
  - Advocates for Youth: www.advocatesforyouth.org
  Runaway Youth/Youth Abscondence:
  - National Runaway Safeline: www.1800runaway.org, 1-800-786-2929

Resources for Health Care Providers
- Futures without Violence: www.futureswithoutviolence.org, www.ipvhealth.org
- Role of the Pediatrician in Youth Violence Prevention[64]

---

there are several limitations to a universal screening approach. Several brief IPV screening instruments have been validated among adult IPV survivors; a brief ARA screening instrument shows promise but has not been assessed in clinical care.[42,43] No studies to date have evaluated the efficacy of a universal screening approach to identify ARA victimization, connect adolescents to resources, or improve health outcomes in clinical care settings. Studies assessing adult IPV screening suggest that such screenings identify only a small number of survivors, thus limiting opportunities to support survivors to those choosing to disclose IPV at a health care visit.[44] Should providers implement universal screening, they should consider that screening alone, without ARA education, or the provision of a resource list in response to a positive screen do not appear to improve outcomes for adult survivors.[45,46] Universal screening in conjunction with universal education may equip survivors with information that can facilitate resource access later.

Indicator-based assessment
Because ARA impacts multiple domains of health, indicators of ARA during a health care visit (see **Box 1**) may vary broadly and may also occur in response to other traumatic experiences or physical health issues. Thus, when present, indicators should prompt consideration for ARA as part of a broad differential diagnosis. Providers may directly address possible ARA in the context of indicators (see **Box 4**). If the adolescent does not disclose ARA, providers may consider sharing information about resources using a universal education approach to facilitate resource access after the

Box 4
Recommended language and scripts

Confidentiality
Before we begin, I want to make sure you know that you can use the resources I'll share with you no matter what you choose to share with me today. But if part of your story is that you're in a relationship with someone who is hurting you or you have questions about if something is ok in a relationship, I'm here to listen if you want to talk. Sometimes when I'm talking to teens about relationships, they share that someone is physically or sexually hurting them or that they're thinking about hurting themselves. When that happens, I need to talk to others to help make sure that young person is safe. That might include a parent or another caregiver, law enforcement, or others. If I need to do this, I let that young person know who I'll be talking to and give choices about how that happens when I can. My main goal is to make sure that young person is safe.

Universal Education
I've started sharing this information with all of my patients because relationships impact things like health and how teens do in school. It includes information about healthy relationships and resources for teens who may be in abusive relationships or just need help navigating complicated relationships. I want you to have this info in case you ever need it for yourself or to help a friend. This is something you can talk with me about, too, but you can use the resources I'm sharing no matter what you choose to share with me today.

Indicator-based Assessment
When patients ask for a pregnancy test, I always check a couple things to make sure that I provide the right resources. Is being pregnant right now something that you want? . . . What are you using for birth control? . . . Some teens have shared with me that it's hard to use condoms or birth control because their partner doesn't want them to do these things. But everyone deserves to be with someone that respects their decisions about using condoms or birth control. How does your partner feel about condoms or birth control?
When patients are having problems with [symptom, for example, headaches, abdomen pain, etc.], I also check in about stress. We know that stress can impact the way our bodies feel. Stressful or traumatic experiences can be related to things like headaches or abdominal pain. Some of the stressful experiences teens share with me are being in a relationship where they're abused or not respected, schoolwork stress, or challenges at home. If these or other stressors are ever part of your experience, I'm here if you want to talk about them. I can share some resources that might help [pause for response].
I always provide information about relationship resources when a patient experiences [ARA indicator] so that they have it in case they ever need it and so they can share it with friends who may need it.

Response to Disclosure (Victimization and Perpetration)
Validation:
• You are not alone and you are not to blame.
• You do not deserve to be treated this way.
• You have courage.
• You have choices.
• You can make your own decisions.
• You are welcome here anytime.
Warm hand-off to resources:
• I'd like to connect you to someone who knows a lot about dealing with challenging or complex relationships. They've helped a lot of teens. You can talk to them today about resources and options and make a plan for what you think might be most helpful for you.

When Mandatory Reporting is Indicated
Based on what you shared, I'm concerned about your safety. Remember how we talked about situations where if a young person is being harmed, I would need to get others involved? This is one of those times that I need to do that to help keep you safe. [share next specific step, for example, talking to parent or social worker].

Safety Planning
• Are you worried you might be in immediate danger?

- Has your partner threatened to kill themselves or you?
- What have you already done to stay safe?
- Do you have a code word to let a friend or trusted adult know you need help?
- Can you stay out of places where you might get trapped?
- What could make getting to school or work safer?
- Who can you let know when you're going to be spending time or alone with your partner? Is calling the police an option for you if you need help right away?
- Do you have a cell phone? Is it possible to keep it charged and with you all the time?
- Does your partner have access to a weapon or a gun?
- If living with a partner: Are you afraid to go home? Do you have a place to go if you need to get away from your house quickly? Can you stash a bag with the things you would need if you needed to leave right away?

visit. Care must be taken to clearly communicate a universal education approach, so adolescents do not perceive resource information provision as a sign of distrust or judgment (see **Box 4**).

Response to disclosure of adolescent relationship abuse victimization and perpetration

The primary aim of response to adolescent disclosure of ARA in health care settings is to validate the disclosure and facilitate connection to resources (see **Box 4**). Health care providers should understand their biases to facilitate an appropriately supportive response. Providers should avoid assumptions and use inclusive language, especially around gender and sexuality and including preferred pronouns. Privacy is essential to building trust and a sense of safety. The provider should believe and validate the adolescent experience and acknowledge any injustice.

A warm hand-off to resources includes a direct connection to a social worker or victim services advocate at the time of disclosure.[4] A shared decision-making approach to resource provision is an important component of survivor-centered care. The adolescent ARA survivor is the expert in their own lived experience and providers should offer resources and safety planning as choices rather than dictating which resources should be used unless there are acute safety concerns or mandated reporting is necessary. This approach promotes adolescent autonomy and may further facilitate adolescent trust in their individual health care provider as well as the health care system as a whole. More details about additional components of response to disclosure (eg, caregiver notification, mandatory reporting) are given in the following paragraphs.

As part of the resources discussed after disclosure, providers should consider offering point-of-care services that may minimize negative sexual and reproductive health outcomes of ARA. These may include time-sensitive services (eg, emergency contraception), as well as other harm reduction resources or health services such as STI testing and treatment, hormonal contraception, or condoms. See **Table 2** for additional health care needs after disclosure.

For adolescents disclosing ARA perpetration, health care providers can validate the disclosure, acknowledging that relationships can be challenging but that respect is always an essential component of healthy and strong relationships. To date, few interventions have been designed that specifically address ARA perpetration. Real Talk, a 30-min motivational interviewing intervention, shows promise to reduce ARA perpetration over time.[47] SafERteens, an emergency department-based intervention for adolescents indicating past 3-month aggressive behavior on a brief screening instrument, shows promise for reducing ARA as well as general peer violence.[48,49]

Table 2
Health care and social needs in response to ARA disclosure[63]

	Immediate[a]	Short-Term	Long-Term
All Adolescents	• Time-sensitive medical needs[b] • Safety planning and danger assessment	• Mental, physical health care • Ongoing safety	• Ongoing health and healing
Immigration or Refugee Considerations	• Interpretation services • Legal services	• Language assistance • Legal services • Immigration relief	• Language classes • Legal services • Family reunification and community
Emancipated Adolescents	• Emergency financial assistance and basic needs (eg, housing) • Legal services	• Employment/income • Legal services	• Career and education

[a] Mandatory reporting may be required depending on disclosure type (eg, physical or sexual abuse) and safety concerns.
[b] May include physical and/or sexual assault injuries, reproductive and sexual health harm reduction (STI testing/treatment, emergency contraception), and mental health concerns (depression, anxiety, and suicidal ideation).

Online resources for adolescents may also be helpful to provide and reinforce healthy relationship behaviors and counter gender norms that create risk for ARA (eg, the Cool-Not Cool game on www.thatsnotcool.com).

Mandatory reporting
Child protective services reporting may be mandated for some forms of ARA. Unfortunately, every state is different with regards to mandatory reporting requirements for ARA (www.childwelfare.gov/topics/systemwide/laws-policies/state/). Many states require that a provider reports physical harm and sexual abuse for anyone who is under the age of 18, with no exemption for ARA. The age of sexual consent also varies by state, with consideration for age gaps between the individuals having sexual intercourse. To maintain patient-provider trust, providers should inform adolescents when mandated reporting is required, providing opportunity for choice when possible (see **Box 4**).

Engaging parents and trusted adults
Parents and other trusted adults can serve as important supports to help reinforce healthy relationship skills. Parental monitoring is a protective factor for adolescent risk behavior in general, as well as for ARA.[50,51] Parent-adolescent conversations about dating and relationships, parental limit-setting around dating, and parental awareness of their adolescent's dating activity comprise parental monitoring around ARA. However, evidence suggests that although many parents talk to their adolescents about dating in general, they do not discuss ARA.[52] Further, parents may be less likely to discuss ARA with their adolescents than topics such as schoolwork, substance use, family finances, and sex.[52] Health care providers have opportunity to encourage open communication between parents and adolescents around dating and relationships. Both adolescents and parents agree that this is an important topic for the adolescent's provider to address.[35]

Parents and other trusted adults can also be a critical resource and ongoing support for adolescents who have experienced ARA. Both adolescents and parents find it acceptable to notify a parent after any type of ARA is disclosed, although evidence suggests this may be less acceptable among adolescents who have experienced ARA.[53] Providers should be sensitive to the potential for parental notification about ARA to have a negative outcome. Shared decision-making that includes exploration and validation of adolescent concerns can enable providers and adolescents to reach a consensus about trusted adult notification. With adolescent permission, providers can help to facilitate difficult conversations between an adolescent and a trusted adult for ongoing support and access to resources. Choices can be offered in this situation; for example, the adolescent may prefer that the provider share about the disclosure without the adolescent being present and then bring the parent and adolescent together to discuss next steps, to tell their parent themselves with the provider present, or for the provider to tell the parent with the adolescent present.

Environmental cues

Posters, pamphlets, hotline cards, and other environmental cues in waiting rooms, examination rooms, or bathrooms may provide an additional opportunity for adolescents experiencing ARA to access resources in the absence of disclosure.

Documentation

Clinical documentation of ARA is important to communicate treatment of physical, mental, and social health care needs but confidentiality must be considered. Health care providers and institutions should establish electronic health record systems, policies, and procedures that accommodate confidentiality needs related to minor adolescents and comply with the requirements for state and federal laws.[54] ARA documentation specifically can include provided medical care, referrals, and safety planning. Careful documentation may also aid police prosecution, should this be desired. Documentation may include photographs of injuries. Clinical documentation should avoid legal terms and phrases that imply doubt.[55]

Adolescent relationship abuse prevention beyond health care settings

Multiple efforts within communities may provide layers of opportunity to support healthy adolescent dating relationships and connect youth in need to ARA resources. Many states have enacted policies mandating that schools provide education on ARA and/or sexual and reproductive health. There is, however, considerable variation in the content of such legislation, which may or may not specify how schools should deliver such education (ie, use of evidence-based programs) or allocate funds toward ARA programming.[56] Further, evidence suggests that the presence of laws mandating school-based ARA education is not associated with reduced victimization.[57] Health care providers can advocate within their municipal community and/or at the state and federal levels to promote the use of available effective school-based ARA prevention programs and allocation of funding to support implementation of such programs.[32,58,59] They may also advocate to ensure that school-based reproductive and sexual health curricula address healthy relationship behaviors and ARA. Additionally, providers may partner with other community organizations, such as churches, youth clubs, or sports teams, to support healthy relationships and offer connections to ARA resources. The Centers for Disease Control and Prevention provides multi-level programs, policies, and practices that can be applied within health care and across other community settings to address ARA[60] as well as youth violence more broadly.[61] These recommendations include engaging influential adults and peers, disrupting developmental pathways toward partner violence, strengthening economic supports for families, and supporting survivors to increase safety and lessen harms.[61] Community-level programming should identify and actively build on community strengths in partnership with community shareholders to ensure that the unique strengths, needs, and culture of the community are considered.

SUMMARY

In conclusion, ARA is common and has a wide range of negative physical, emotional, and psychosocial consequences. Health care providers can use a healing-centered, multidisciplinary approach across all levels of ARA prevention to promote healthy relationships and connect adolescents to the health treatment and advocacy services that they need.

CLINICS CARE POINTS

- ARA may include one or more types of abusive behaviors, including physical, sexual, emotional, cyber, or economic abuse, reproductive coercion, and transactional sex.

- Youth experiencing ARA may not feel comfortable sharing this during a healthcare visit. A universal education approach that provides all youth with information on healthy relationships and resources for ARA provides opportunity for youth to access resources regardless of disclosure.

- To promote adolescent-provider trust and enable youth to make an informed disclosure of ARA, providers should share limits of confidentiality before addressing ARA.

- Providers should understand their state legislation regarding mandated reporting.

- A survivor-centered response to ARA disclosure includes validation and shared decision-making with the adolescent about resources and supports, including a warm hand-off to victim services resources and connection to a trusted adult.

- Providers should address both immediate and long-term health needs and ongoing support after ARA disclosure.

CONFLICTS OF INTEREST

The authors have no conflicts of interest to declare.

DISCLOSURES

This work was supported by the Eunice Kennedy Shriver National Institute of Child Health & Human Development (K23HD098299, K.A. Randell) and the Centers for Disease Control and Prevention (K01CE003326–01–00, L. Jarvis). The content is solely the responsibility of the authors and does not necessarily represent the official views of the National Institutes of Health or the Centers for Disease Control and Prevention.

REFERENCES

1. Basile KC, Clayton HB, DeGue S, et al. Interpersonal violence victimization among high school students - Youth Risk Behavior Survey, United States, 2019. MMWR (Morb Mortal Wkly Rep) 2020;69(1):28–37.
2. Leemis RW, Friar N, Khatiwada S, et al. The national intimate partner and sexual violence Survey: 2016/2017 report on intimate partner violence. Atlanta, GA: National Center for Injury Prevention and Control, Centers for Disease Control and Prevention; 2022.
3. Sardinha L, Maheu-Giroux M, Stockle H, et al. Global, regional, and national prevalence estimates of physical or sexual, or both, intimate partner violence against women in 2018. Lancet 2022;399(10327):803–13.

4. Miller E, Levenson RR. Hanging out or Hooking up: clinical Guidelines on responding to adolescent relationship abuse. Futures Without Violence; 2013.
5. Caridade S, Braga T, Borrajo E. Cyber dating abuse (CDA): Evidence from a systematic review. Aggress Violent Behav 2019;48:152–68.
6. Rothman EF, Bazzi AR, Bair-Merritt MH. "I'll do whatever as long as you keep telling me that I'm important": a case study illustrating the link between adolescent dating violence and sex trafficking victimization. J Appl Res Child 2015; 6(1–21).
7. Anderson PM, Coyle KK, Johnson A, et al. An exploratory study of adolescent pimping relationships. J Prim Prev 2014;35(2):113–7.
8. Reed SM, Kennedy MA, Decker MR, et al. Friends, family, and boyfriends: An analysis of relationship pathways into commercial sexual exploitation. Child Abuse Negl 2019;90:1–12.
9. Myhill A, Hohl K. The "Golden Thread": Coercive Control and Risk Assessment for Domestic Violence. J Interpers Violence 2019;34(21–22):4477–97.
10. Taylor BG, Mumford EA. A national descriptive portrait of adolescent relationship abuse: results from the National Survey on Teen Relationships and Intimate Violence. J Interpers Violence 2016;31(6). 963-988.
11. Reyes HLM, Foshee VA, Niolon PH, et al. Gender role attitudes and male adolescent dating violence perpetration: Normative beliefs as moderators. J Youth Adolesc 2016;45(2):350–60.
12. Northridge JL, Silver EJ, Talib HJ, et al. Reproductive coercion in high school-aged girls: Associations with reproductive health risk and intimate partner violence. J Pediatr Adolesc Gynecol 2017;30(6):603–8.
13. Espelage D, Merrin G, Hatchel T. Peer victimization and dating violence among LGBTQ youth: The impact of school violence and crime on mental health outcomes. Youth Violence and Juvenile Justcie 2018;16(2):156–73.
14. Martin-Storey A, Pollitt AM, Baams L. Profiles and predictors of dating violence among sexual and gender minority adolescents. J Adolesc Health 2020;68(6): 1155–61.
15. Silverman JG, Raj A, Mucci LA, et al. Dating violence against adolescent girls and associated substance use, unhealthy weight control, sexual risk behavior, pregnancy, and suicidality. JAMA 2001;286(5):572–9.
16. Miller E, McCauley HL, Tancredi DJ, et al. Recent reproductive coercion and unintended pregnancy among female family planning clients. Contraception 2014; 89:122–8.
17. Exner-Cortens D, Eckenrode J, Rothman E. Longitudinal associations between teen dating violence victimization and adverse health outcomes. Pediatrics 2013;131(1):71–8.
18. Foshee V, Reyes H, Gottfredson N, et al. A longitudinal examination of psychological, behavioral, adademic and relationship consequences of dating abuse victimization among a primarily rural sample of adolescents. J Adolesc Health 2013;53(6):729–32.
19. Teitelman AM, Ratcliffe SJ, Morales-Aleman MM, et al. Sexual relationship power, intimate partner violence, and condom use among minority urban girls. J Interpers Violence 2008;23(12):1684–712.
20. Goldstein AL, Walton MA, Cunningham RM, et al. Correlates of gambling among youth in an inner-city emergency department. Psychol Addict Behav 2009;23(1): 113–21.
21. Adhia A, Kernic MA, Hemenway D, et al. Intimate partner homicide of adolescents. JAMA Pediatr 2019;173(6):571–7.

22. Balocchini E, Chiamenti G, Lamborghini A. Adolescents: Which risks for their life and health? J Prev Med Hyg 2013;54(4):191–4.

23. National Academies of Sciences, Engineering, and Medicine, Health and Medicine Division, Division of behavioral and Social Sciences and Education, Board on Children, Youth, and Families, Committee on the Neurobiological and Socio-Behavioral Science of Adolescent Development and its Applications. In: Backes EP, Bonnie RJ, editors. The Promise of adolescence: Realizing Opportunity for all youth. Washington (DC): National Academies Press (US); 2019.

24. Reaching Teens: Strength-Based, Trauma-Sensitive. In: Ginsburgh KR, Brett Z, McClain R, editors. Resilience-building communication strategies Rooted in positive youth development. 2nd edition. American Academy of Pediatrics; 2020.

25. Miller E. Healing-Centered Engagement: Fostering Connections Rather than Forcing Disclosures. In: Ginsburgh KR, Brett Z, McClain R, editors. Reaching teens: Strength-based, trauma-sensitive, resilience-building communication strategies Rooted in positive youth development. American Academy of Pediatrics; 2020.

26. Ginwright S. The future of healing: Shifting from trauma informed care to healing centered engagement. Medium. Updated May 31, 2018, https://ginwright.medium.com/the-future-of-healing-shifting-from-trauma-informed-care-to-healing-centered-engagement-634f557ce69c. Accessed 21 May/2021.

27. Crenshaw K. Mapping the margins: Intersectionality, identity politics, and violence against women of color. Stanford Law Rev 1991;43(6):1241–99.

28. The Social-Ecological Model: A Framework for Prevention. National Center for Injury Prevention and Control, Division of Violence Prevention. Updated January 18, 2022. Accessed February 27, 2023, https://www.cdc.gov/violenceprevention/about/social-ecologicalmodel.html.

29. Dank M, Lachman P, Zweig JM, et al. Dating violence experiences of lesbian, gay, bisexual, and transgender youth. J Youth Adolesc 2014;43(5):846–57.

30. Padilla-Medina DM, Williams JR, Ravi K, et al. Teen dating violence help-seeking intentions and behaviors among ethnically and racially diverse youth: A systematic review. Trauma Violence Abuse 2021. 1524838020985569.

31. Ragavan MI, Syed-Swift Y, Elwy AR, et al. The influence of culture on healthy relationship formation and teen dating violence: A qualitative analysis of South Asian female youth residing in the United States. J Interpers Violence 2021;36(7–8): NP4336–62.

32. Preventing multiple forms of violence: a strategic vision for connecting the Dots. Atlanta, GA: Division of Violence Prevention, National Center for Injury Prevention and Control, Centers for Disease Control and Prevention; 2016.

33. Lewis-O'Connor A, Warren A, Lee JV, et al. The state of the science on trauma injury. Womens Health 2019. 1745506519861234.

34. Violence Prevention Fundamentals. Centers for Disease Control and Prevention. Updated July 22, 2019, https://vetoviolence.cdc.gov/apps/main/prevention-information/47. Accessed February 27, 2023.

35. Tiffany-Appleton S, Mickievicz E, Ortizay Y, et al. Adolescent relationship abuse prevention in pediatric primary care: Provider, adolescent, and parent perspectives. Acad Pediatr 2022. S1976-2859(22)0063307.

36. Bundock K, Chan C, Hewitt O. Adolescents' help-seeking behavior and intentions followign adolescent dating violence: A systematic review. Trauma Violence Abuse 2020;21(2):350–66.

37. Miller E, Goldstein S, McCauley HL, et al. A school health center intervention for abusive adolescent relationships: a cluster RCT. Pediatrics 2015;135(1):76–85.

38. Hill A L, Jones KA, McCauley HL, et al. Reproductive coercion and relationship abuse among adolescents and yougn women seeking care at school health centers. Obstet Gynecol 2019;134(2):351–9.

39. Miller E, McCauley HL, Decker MR, et al. Implementation of a family planning clinic-based partner violence and reproductive coercion intervention: Provider and patient perspectives. Perspect Sex Reprod Health 2017;49(2):85–93.

40. Hanging Out or Hooking Up: Teen safety card. Futures Without Violence. Accessed February 27, 2023, Available at: https://www.futureswithoutviolence.org/hanging-out-or-hooking-up-teen-safety-card/.

41. U.S. Preventive Services Taskforce. Screening for intimate partner violence, elder abuse, and abuse of vulnerable adults. JAMA 2018;320(16):1678–87.

42. Rabin RF, Jennings JM, Campbell JC, et al. Intimate partner violence screening tools: a systematic review. Am J Prev Med 2009;36(5):439–45.e4.

43. Rothman EF, Campbell JK, Bair-Mertitt M, et al. Validity of a three-item dating abuse victimization screening tool in a 11–21 year old sample. BMC Pediatr 2022;22:337.

44. Litzau M, Dowd MD, Miller MK, et al. Universal intimate partner violence in the pediatric emergency department and urgent care setting: a retrospective review. Pediatr Emerg Care 2020;36(12):e686–9.

45. Klevens J, Kee R, Trick W, et al. Effect of screening for partner violence on women's quality of life. JAMA 2012;308(7):681–9.

46. MacMillan HL, Wathen CN, Jamieson E, et al. Screening for intimate partner violence in health care settings: a randomized trial. JAMA 2009;302(5):493–501.

47. Rothman EF, Stuart GL, Heeren T, et al. The effects of a health care-based brief intervention on dating abuse perpetration: Results of a randomized controlled trial. Prev Sci 2020;21(3):366–76.

48. Carter PM, Cunningham RM, Eisman AB, et al. Translating violence prevention programs from research to practice: SafERteens implementation in an urban emergency department. J Emerg Med 2022;62(1):109–24.

49. Cunningham RM, Whiteside L, Chermack ST, et al. Dating violence: outcomes following a brief motivational interviewing intervention among at-risk adolescents in an urban emergency department. Acad Emerg Med 2013;20(6):562–9.

50. Davis J, Ports K, Basile KC, et al. Understanding the buffering effects of protective factors on the relationship between adverse childhood experiences and teen dating violence perpetration. J Youth Adolesc 2019;48(12):2343–59.

51. Khetarpal SK, Szoko N, Culyba AJ, et al. Associations between parental monitoring and mutliple types of youth violence victimization: A brief report. J Interpers Violence 2021;37:19–20.

52. Rothman EF, Miller E, Terpeluk A, et al. The proportion of U.S. parents who talk with their adolescent children about dating abuse. J Adolesc Health 2011;49:216–8.

53. Wiebelhaus JN, Miller MK, Sherman AK, et al. Adolescent and parent perspectives on confidentiality after adolescent relationship abuse disclosure. J Adolesc Health 2020. S1054-139X(20)30595-4.

54. Confidentiality in Adolescent Health Care: ACOG Committee Opinion, Number 803. Obstet Gynecol 2020;135(4):e171–7.

55. Rudman WJ. Coding and documentation of domestic violence. Family Violence Prevention Fund; 2000. Accessed February 28, 2023. https://www.futureswithoutviolence.org/userfiles/file/HealthCare/codingpaper.pdf.

56. Adhia A, Kray M, Bowen D, et al. Assessment of variation in US state laws addressing the prevention of and response to teen dating violence in secondary schools. JAMA Pediatr 2022;176(8):797–803.
57. Harland KK, Vakkalanka JP, Peek-Asa C, et al. State-level teen dating violence education laws and teen dating violence victimisation in the USA: a cross-sectional analysis of 36 states. Inj Prev 2020. injuryprev-2020-043657.
58. Preventing Teen Dating Violence, https://youth.gov/youth-topics/teen-dating-violence/prevention. Accessed February 27, 2023.
59. Dating Matters. National Center for Injury Prevention and Control, Division of Violence Prevention. Updated August 3, 2018, https://www.cdc.gov/violenceprevention/intimatepartnerviolence/datingmatters/index.html. Accessed February 27, 2023.
60. Niolon PH, Kearns M, Dills J, et al. Preventing intimate partner violence across the Lifespan: a Technical Package of programs, policies, and practices. National Center for Injury Prevention and Control, Centers for Disease Control and Prevention; 2017.
61. David-Ferdon C, Vivolo-Kantor AM, Dahlberg LL, et al. A Comprehensive Technical Package for the prevention of youth violence and associated risk behaviors. National Center for Injury Prevention and Control, Centers for Disease Control and Prevention; 2016.
62. Teen Power and Control Wheel. Family Crisis Center, https://familycrisis centeriowa.org/teen-dating/teen-power-control-wheel/. Accessed February 27, 2023.
63. Human Trafficking and Health Care. The National Health Collaborative on Violence and Abuse, http://nhcva.org/files/2018/03/PDF_Trafficking-_Slides_Part_II.pdf. Accessed February 28, 2023.
64. Committee on Injury, Violence, and Poison Prevention. Role of the Pediatrician in Youth Violence Prevention. Pediatrics 2009;124(1):393–402.

Assault Injury and Community Violence

Uma Raman, MD[a], Edouard Coupet II, MD, MS[b],
James Dodington, MD[c],*

KEYWORDS

- Community violence • Assaultive injuries
- Hospital-based violence intervention programs • Trauma-informed care
- Place-based trauma interventions

KEY POINTS

- Community violence happens between unrelated individuals, who may or may not know each other, generally outside the home, and often results in assaultive injuries.
- Community violence interventions can prevent assaultive injuries and assist victims of community violence. These include, as key examples, hospital-based violence intervention programs, violence interrupter or street outreach programs, group violence intervention programs, and community place-based interventions.
- Trauma-informed care, described as a practice of encouraging health care providers to consider the physical and psychological impact of trauma when treating patients, is foundational to the success of community violence intervention.
- Place-based environmental interventions, such as green-space rehabilitation, can decrease community violence on the population level, and further research and developments are needed in this area.
- Substance use is a significant barrier to intervention program involvement and greater research and program development is needed to support substance use treatment of those impacted by community violence.

INTRODUCTION

Community violence happens between unrelated individuals, who may or may not know each other, generally outside the home. Examples include assaultive injuries (eg, stabbing or a physical fight) and/or firearm injuries among individuals or groups in communities inclusive of schools and on the streets. Research indicates that youth

[a] Pediatric Critical Care, Yale New Haven Hospital, Yale School of Medicine, 100 York Street, Suite 1F, New Haven, CT 06511, USA; [b] Yale School of Medicine, Core Faculty, Addiction Medicine, 464 Congress Avenue, Suite 260, New Haven, CT 06890, USA; [c] Yale School of Medicine, Yale New Haven Center for Injury and Violence Prevention, 100 York Street, Suite 1F, New Haven, CT 06511, USA
* Corresponding author.
E-mail address: James.dodington@yale.edu

Pediatr Clin N Am 70 (2023) 1103–1114
https://doi.org/10.1016/j.pcl.2023.06.007
pediatric.theclinics.com

and young adults (ages 10–34), particularly those in communities of color, and low socioeconomic status/poverty are disproportionately impacted for reasons involving systemic racism and disinvestment.[1] Evidence-based community violence intervention strategies can prevent community violence in youth and assist those already injured.

The US Department of Justice defines the community violence intervention approach as a strategy that uses one or more of the following:

1. Trusted credible messengers to implement key intervention components
2. Partnerships with representatives of affected communities in the development, implementation, and augmentation of a particular strategy
3. Input of the private, public, and community stakeholders most impacted by violence
4. Data that are vetted for racial, ethnic, economic, and other biases
5. Practices that are informed by and respond to the trauma endured by historically underinvested communities
6. The principles of racial, socioeconomic, and ethnic equity

Community violence interventions should be centered around community needs; use evidence and data to inform practices; be inclusive; and demonstrate impact through reduction of violence and/or improvement in patient-centered outcomes, trauma symptoms, and reintegration of trauma victims into the community.[2,3]

In this article, we discuss hospital-based violence intervention programs (HVIPs), street outreach or violence interrupter programs, group violence intervention (GVI), school-based counseling partnership, and a brief description of place-based violence interventions. Of note, after stabilization and discharge from the hospital injured youth and young adults may require specialized medical care that is difficult for patients' families to coordinate on their own. In the short term, patients may return to the emergency department (ED) or trauma surgery clinics for wound checks, ostomy care, drain removal, and pain management, although these settings can be retraumatizing.[4,5] These safety-net resources may facilitate connection to preventive care, risk reduction counseling, case management, and trauma-focused support.[6]

Trauma-informed care serves as a critical underpinning for these interventions. It is briefly discussed in this article and addressed more fully in other sections of this issue. The importance of a collaborative ecosystem of interventions/programs as described previously to address community violence cannot be overemphasized.

PATIENT CASE

Kai was 14 years old when he was found unconscious in a car after being shot seven times in the chest, abdomen, and back. He arrived at a trauma center in severe hemorrhagic shock requiring multiple transfusions. He went on to require endotracheal intubation, bilateral chest tubes, and an emergent thoracotomy and exploratory laparotomy to achieve hemostasis. Bowel resection was not required. After several days in the pediatric intensive care unit, he was extubated and ultimately awoke but found that he could not feel or move his lower extremities. MRI findings noted one of the bullet paths to be close to the spine, increasing suspicion for spinal injury. This would leave him indefinitely paralyzed from the waist down.

Kai left the hospital with intact cardiac, respiratory, and abdominal function but sustained paraplegia. He required intensive inpatient rehabilitation and aggressive pain management in the setting of his spinal injury and deconditioning from prolonged pediatric intensive care unit hospitalization. Additional stressors include significant emotional and psychological trauma from the event itself and his medical care, adjustment to altered function, and barriers to remaining on track at school. Kai's family also endured trauma from this event and the stress of adjusting to his new medical needs. Finally, it was unknown who shot Kai and for what reason, creating barriers in seeking justice and raising fear about their collective safety in their neighborhood.

Having identified Kai's complex needs, we now discuss the various interventions available and then review how these interventions specifically may help address those needs.

HOSPITAL-BASED INTERVENTION PROGRAMS

HVIPs are multidisciplinary hospital-based programs that combine the efforts of medical providers with trusted community-based partners to provide intensive case management through trauma-informed care to patients who have suffered assaultive injuries. HVIPs in the United States were first organized by the founding members of the National Network of Hospital-based Violence Intervention Programs, now known as the Health Alliance for Violence Intervention (https://www.thehavi.org/). There are now more than 50 programs across the United States, including the initial programs in Boston, Baltimore, Newark, Oakland, Philadelphia, San Francisco, and Milwaukee.

An HVIP typically consists of medical professionals, social workers, and violence prevention professionals (VPPs). The VPPs, or trauma-intervention specialists, are often members of the local communities they serve and are trained in trauma-informed care acting as credible messengers for the program. Many people who have suffered violent injuries are distrustful of health care institutions, and VPPs are specially trained to break through this distrust and provide victims services and intensive case management. These highly trained paraprofessionals, some former victims of community violence themselves, can quickly engage violently injured patients and their families during or after the hospital setting for the patient.

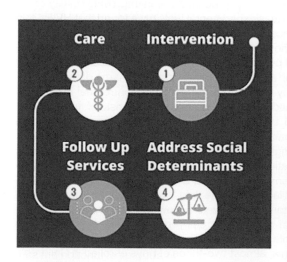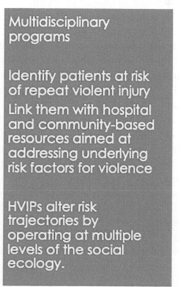

Fig. 1. Hospital-based Violence Intervention Program Care Diagram. (*Courtesy of* the Health Alliance for Violence Intervention.)

Although each hospital or health system may have unique resources and practices, HVIPs share the same general approach (**Fig. 1**). The patient is approached by VPPs during or soon after their contact with the medical system for an injury related to assault. This is considered "the golden opportunity" for intervention. After gaining trust and introducing the program, VPPs may connect the family to a core violence intervention team that can include the VPP, various supervisors, and a mental health professional. This team works with clients and their families to develop a postdischarge plan that meets their immediate safety needs, provides critical psychosocial services, and establishes mutually derived goals that focus on healing and recovery. They then connect the family with resources that can address the various unique social needs that arise as the patient returns to the community, such as rehabilitation, medical follow-up, school accommodations, and grief counseling. The team also attends to basic, concrete needs that address social determinants of health, such as food insecurity, safe housing, and transportation (see **Fig. 1**). A mental health clinician on the team can provide therapeutic interventions, such as psychoeducational acute counseling, following with outpatient therapy services. This form of intensive case management promotes survivors' physical and mental recovery while also improving their social and economic conditions. A focus on patient-centered outcomes and goal-based achievement is central to implementation and evaluation of HVIPs, endorsed by program leaders and victims alike.[7,8]

Some programs have additional features that have evolved from patient and family needs. For example, the Violence Intervention Program at Children's Hospital of Philadelphia offers not only embedded mental health care but also legal advocacy. Healing Hurt People at St. Christopher's Hospital for Children in Philadelphia offers the Safety, Emotions, Loss, Future (SELF) curriculum, which helps patients develop insight into trauma and self-regulatory skills.[9] Some programs also offer training in trauma-informed care to the medical staff in the ED and inpatient settings. Programmatic follow-up postdischarge varies between programs and participants within a program, but most programs aim for at least 4 to 6 months of follow-up; some offer a minimum follow-up of 1 year.

Evidence suggests that these programs can be effective in improving quality of life and reducing reinjury. Additionally, quasiexperimental trials have found that HVIPs had benefits in decreasing juvenile justice involvement.[10] One study of Boston's Violence Intervention Advocacy Program showed a decrease in the overall number of penetrating injuries caused by violence presenting to the Boston Medical Center ED over the 12 years of Violence Intervention Advocacy Program postdischarge data. In particular, pediatric injuries decreased by 53%.[11] One randomized control trial in Chicago showed that HVIP participants had a 60% decrease in their risk of future injury compared with nonparticipants (8.1% vs 20.3%).[12] A similar program in Baltimore showed a 15% decrease (5% of participants vs 20.3% of nonparticipants).[13]

HVIP participation has wide-ranging benefits beyond reinjury. Given that violent injury is a psychologically traumatic event, these programs are well-equipped to address signs and symptoms of emotional trauma and posttraumatic stress. Up to 75% of patients who enroll in Philadelphia's Healing Hurt People Program experienced posttraumatic stress symptoms.[9] A 10-year review of San Francisco's Wraparound Project found that 51% of participants self-reported mental health needs, 85% of which the program was able to address.[14] In one study for pediatric patients at Children's Hospital of Philadelphia, almost two-thirds of boys enrolled in Children's Hospital of Philadelphia VIP had clinically significant Post Traumatic Stress Symptoms (PTSS), and 89% self-identified at least one mental health need to be addressed as part of the case management.[15] Mental health and emotional needs were also identified as paramount outcome domains as defined by a consensus study of HVIP directors and frontline workers using a Delphi technique to prioritize important outcomes for HVIPs.[7]

VIOLENCE INTERRUPTION AND STREET OUTREACH

Violence interruption programs use members of the community as mentors and points of contact for high-risk youth and young adults. The first program was started in Chicago by Dr Gary Slutkin at the University of Illinois. Baltimore was next to adopt a similar program in 2007. There are now violence interruption programs across the United States, in such cities as New York, Tucson, and Richmond (California). The programs typically use the following strategies: interrupt violence through conflict mediation; change the trajectory of potential perpetrators through intensive, mentor-led cognitive behavioral therapy; connect high-risk youth to community resources; and change group norms around violence through public education/community events.[16] Violence interrupters or "street outreach workers" are usually members of the same communities in which they work and are trained in trauma-informed care and violence interruption. They go into their communities and reach out to high-risk youth to provide supportive relationships and connect youth to resources for such needs as substance use, violence, court involvement, and mental health. Street outreach workers remain in neighborhoods in the evenings and nights to respond to critical incidents and mediate conflicts as they arise. Some programs incorporate an immediate trauma response team, which goes to the site of an incident or hospital to aid victims and reduce the risk of retaliation.

The most extensively studied violence interruption programs are in Chicago, Baltimore, and Brooklyn. Sections of Chicago saw a substantial decrease in violence in areas where the Cure Violence program was implemented, and a concomitant increase in violence in those same areas when funding was cut from the program.[17] When Baltimore Safe Streets, a violence-interrupter program, was implemented, three of the four neighborhoods saw a 56% decrease in homicides and a 34% decrease in nonfatal shootings over a 3-year period.[17] The violence interruption program in Brooklyn did not show a significant decrease in violence, showing the difficulty in uniform results across the spectrum of these programs.[17] The reduction of violence was variable between implantation sites, because individual factors, such as community-level buy-in and engagement, did influence the program's impact.[16] Limitations in these studies include barriers to consistent program implementation at maximum capacity and the inability to control for concurrent changes in the neighborhood that may contribute to violence reduction. Programs continue to face challenges with inconsistent funding and high staff turnover, and there is discussion about how to maintain the safety and well-being of violence interrupters who must work in high-risk areas without backup from law enforcement. Finally, given that many violence interrupters are often individuals who were violence-involved at some point, attention needs to be focused on how to reduce vicarious trauma as they process their own emotional trauma.[18]

Further development of the violence interruption models has aimed to address these program challenges and focus on mental health intervention. Rather than relying on location-based outreach and working separately from law enforcement, Roca in Baltimore and Rapid Employment and Development Initiative (READI) in Chicago use law enforcement to identify the highest-risk individuals across the city. Because they gain referrals from law enforcement agencies, they often maintain more consistent clientele and can avoid sending workers to higher-risk areas.[19] Roca has seen success through the implementation of a cognitive-behavioral health intervention carried out by trusted mentors (https://rocainc.org/), and READI combines mental health interventions with career pathway interventions that provide clients with economic empowerment as a means of breaking the cycle of violence (https://www.heartlandalliance.org/readi/).

Other cities have also built hybrid approaches between violence interruption, hospital-based violence prevention, and GVI. Many of these newer models show promise but remain under investigation. One barrier is the large funding stream that must be dedicated to these programs for them to succeed. As the violence interruption strategies continue to evolve, experts acknowledge a need for programs to specifically adapt to changes in social interactions and conflict on social media platforms, a widespread increase in firearm violence, changes in gang culture, and unsafe working conditions for violence interrupters.[19]

GROUP VIOLENCE INTERVENTION

The GVI strategy, also known as focused deterrence or the gun violence reduction strategy, is a law enforcement–based solution that identifies and intervenes with groups of individuals at high risk for violence. Law enforcement personnel partner with social workers, community liaisons affected by gun violence, and community organizations to identify alternatives to help high-risk individuals. As a team, they approach key group violence-involved members and notify them of the potential legal ramifications of any continued activities. The team offers individual resources for lifestyle changes, and the community worker then spends time connecting them to these resources. A systematic review of 24 quasiexperimental studies on focused deterrence found significant reductions in crime, particularly firearm-related violent crimes, in the areas that implemented the program.[20] GVI resulted in a 63% reduction in youth homicides in Boston, a 44% reduction in gun-related assaults in Indianapolis, and significant reductions in violent crime in Los Angeles after the implementation of GVI strategies.[21] These study results are limited by a short period of analysis and a lack of standardized methodology in implementing this intervention.[22] Although GVI research provides a better understanding of the social network of violence exposure, further work is needed in this area. Of note, because of distrust, some communities may find it difficult to apply an intervention that involves law enforcement.

SCHOOL-BASED COUNSELING

Some schools can provide short-term counseling and intervention referral for children who have experienced violence, and act as a liaison to the programs outlined previously. For example, Succeed Boston provides short-term counseling and interventions for children who commit high-risk offenses, such as bringing a weapon to school, along with academic support and social-emotional skill-building opportunities.[11] Although there is limited evidence on efficacy, this is a promising model that can increase access to therapies and services and potentially interface with HVIPs, and interruption programs. Further information on school-based interventions and policies are addressed elsewhere in this issue.

TRAUMA-INFORMED CARE

Trauma-informed care is best described as health care providers and family-serving personnel considering the physical and psychological impact of trauma when treating patients. This is particularly important for victims of assaultive injury. Typical components of this strategy include assessing for signs and symptoms of trauma, optimizing experience in the medical setting to reduce trauma, using deescalation techniques to address stress-related experiences, understanding law enforcement's role in trauma cases, and maintaining knowledge of the resources available for patients.[23] The medical setting can be optimized to reduce trauma by having a single team member as a point person, maintaining a calm atmosphere, reminding patients that they are removed from the site of the incident and emphasizing safety, discussing the care plan with patients, incorporating their wishes where possible to increase a sense of control, making realistic statements regarding positive outcomes, and avoiding statements that exacerbate self-blame.[24] Most trauma-informed care protocols are used In mental health settings, but there is emerging implementation and research on trauma-informed care in the acute care setting. A qualitative assessment of emergency medical providers found that patient and family distrust of providers, interactions with law enforcement, and a lack of clear role in the social-emotional support of trauma patients were barriers to providing trauma-informed care.[24] Further information on trauma-informed care and psychosocial intervention is available in other sections of this issue.

PLACE-BASED PROGRAMMING

There are many programs developed by community members that focus on positive youth development, community rehabilitation, grief counseling after experiencing violence, alternative community-based activities to support nonviolence, and advocacy for the prevention of gun violence. Some of these are collectively called place-based interventions. These population-level interventions aim to enhance safety and decrease crime by making significant physical changes in the community. Such interventions as green-spacing, community garden creation, and repair of buildings and sidewalks have been shown to decrease firearm-related injury and violence in neighborhoods with a history of high rates of community violence. Green-spacing involves cleaning up vacant lots and other neglected spaces and applying low-cut grass and short perimeter fences to create usable communal spaces. A recent study of this intervention in Philadelphia showed reductions in local crime rates, and ongoing efforts are underway in other cities.[25] In Flint, Michigan, streets with maintained vacant lots have had a 40% less violent crime rate than streets with abandoned lots.[26] Importantly, these local, physical improvements could serve as catalyst events for multiple programs to collaborate at a local level, with the potential for significant and long-standing impact.[27,28] Studying the effectiveness of place-based programs in reducing rates of violence must include authentic partnerships between academic and community entities, and funding is needed to sustain the programs and support the research. Reviews of existing literature suggest that place-based programs increase community engagement.[29] Furthermore, multidimensional community prevention programs can reduce assaults and homicides by 40%.[30] Place-based programming continues to be a promising strategy to improve communities through programs developed by those most in touch with the community's needs.

SUBSTANCE USE AND COMMUNITY VIOLENCE VICTIMIZATION

Alcohol and other drug use is a critical modifiable risk factor for community violence. Substance use is widely understood to be a significant risk factor for being a victim and perpetrator of community violence, with alcohol being the most studied substance. Alcohol decreases inhibition and decision-making capacity while increasing aggression. A meta-analysis of 37 EDs in 18 countries determined that 91% of assault-related injuries were attributable to alcohol use.[31] Existing evidence has shown that adolescents who start drinking younger and more frequently are at increased risk for perpetration and victimization of violence.[32] A study of youth firearm homicide victims found that a personal history of alcohol use and living in a neighborhood with high densities of alcohol outlets were both associated with increased odds of firearm homicide deaths.[32] Among other drugs, cocaine, amphetamine-type stimulants, and phencyclidine have also been shown to cause increased aggression and impaired judgement.[33,34] Yet cannabis is the most identified drug in violently injured individuals; although evolving, research surrounding this relationship is notably complex. This relationship is likely related to the physical state of withdrawal, aspects of the illegal drug trade, mutually held risk factors of problem behavior, and the use of drugs to cope with the negative effects of violence (ie, "self-medication"). In addition to increasing the risk of violence, substance use is also associated with worse outcomes including increased risk of reinjury, increased ED visits, and decreased engagement in recovery programs, such as HVIPs.[35–38] Violence prevention programs that incorporate evidence-based strategies to reduce substance use and/or refer to specialty addiction treatment have the potential to decrease program attrition and risk of reinjury.[39–41]

CASE FOLLOW-UP

The medical staff strived to use a trauma-informed approach to understand Kai's physical pain and anxiety during his admission and believed he was a good candidate for the hospital's violence intervention program. Kai and his family were approached by a VPP during his intensive care unit admission. After extensive discussion, Kai was connected with a victim advocate and a mental health professional to form his violence intervention team. His victim advocate helped him navigate setting up inpatient and subsequent outpatient rehabilitation, and outpatient surgical follow-up appointments. They helped the family connect with the school to arrange for continued schoolwork during his rehabilitation, discuss an altered schedule for graduation, and plan for the accommodations required when he returned to school. The victim advocate spoke with the family to determine the safety of their neighborhood and assisted them in exploring options for moving. The mental health professional provided immediate interventions to reduce acute traumatic stress symptoms in the hospital. During inpatient rehabilitation, the violence intervention team continued to check in with Kai and his family.

Once Kai was discharged from the inpatient rehabilitation, his team helped facilitate any additional needed school accommodations and connected Kai and his sibling to trauma-informed therapy in an outpatient setting through a local community-based nonprofit. The school did not offer school-based counseling. They also helped Kai navigate and keep track of all outpatient surgical follow-up appointments and outpatient physical therapy appointments and coordinate care with his primary care provider. Kai's pain regimen was able to be optimized and weaned, and his team ensured he followed up with a pain medicine physician for continued management.

Through therapy, it was found that one of Kai's siblings was trying to learn who shot his brother. He felt significant anger and expressed a desire for retaliation. This sibling was connected with an outreach worker from the local violence interruption initiative for further mentorship and support.

His family remained in the same house, but it was noted that green-spacing initiatives were occurring in the blocks around them. Through the same community-based nonprofit offering therapy to Kai, the family was connected to a family support group.

DISCUSSION

Community violence interventions can best serve youth and young adults when they are developed in partnership with communities; evidence-based; trauma-informed; and founded in the principles of racial, socioeconomic, and ethnic equity. Multiple community violence intervention strategies exist at the level of the hospital, school, and broader community to provide access to therapy/services and support networks for youth who have experienced an assault and those who are at risk of injury. These interventions show promising outcomes for victims and those at risk in terms of emotional well-being and rehabilitation, and reductions in subsequent community violence. Additionally, trauma-informed care is a well-established foundation for all of these programs and can be used to mitigate acute stress in the setting of recent trauma.

Barriers and opportunities for program expansion include consistent funding; access of grassroots or community-based organizations to key infrastructure for data collection and analysis; and consistent community, state, and federal support. Other comorbidities, such as substance use, complicate the implementation of violence prevention strategies and, as a potentially modifiable risk factor, the co-occurrence merits further exploration. Finally, assaultive injury impacting youth and young adults in the United States must be understood in the context of structural racism and historical factors that have led to underinvestment in communities most impacted. Broad coalitions of health care organizations, such as the American College of Surgeons and the American Academy of Pediatrics, have recognized the need to work to address these fundamental roots of community violence.[42,43]

Further investment in and evaluation of community violence intervention programs are important ways that society can facilitate reentry into the community of assault-injured individuals, by improving mental health outcomes, quality of life, and overall well-being. These restorative efforts are likely to play a significant role in breaking the cycle of violence.

CLINICS CARE POINTS

- Clinicians should make every effort to make themselves aware of community-based resources in their practice area for patients who experience assault injuries because of community violence. Intervention programs can prevent assaultive injuries and assist victims of community violence.
- These include hospital-based violence intervention programs, violence interrupter or street outreach programs, and group violence intervention programs.
- Incorporation of trauma-informed care, described as a practice of encouraging health care providers to consider the physical and psychological impact of trauma when treating patients, is foundational to the success of community violence interventions and is important in any aspect of pediatric practice.
- Clinicians should make themselves aware of substance abuse treatment programs in their practice area.

DISCLOSURE

All authors declare no commercial and financial conflicts in the submission of this article.

REFERENCES

1. Community Violence Prevention. Centers for Disease Control and Prevention. Available at: https://www.cdc.gov/violenceprevention/communityviolence/index.html. Published June 8, 2022. Accessed May 7, 2023.
2. Community based violence intervention and prevention initiative (CVIPI): Overview. Bureau of Justice Assistance. Available at: https://bja.ojp.gov/program/community-violence-intervention/overview. Accessed May 7, 2023.
3. Weller BEFS, Ault AK. Youth access to medical homes and medical home components by race and ethnicity. Matern Child Health J 2020 2020;24(2):241–9.
4. Jacoby SFRT, Holena DN, Kaufman EJ. A safe haven for the injured? Urban trauma care at the intersection of healthcare, law enforcement, and race. Soc Sci Med 2018;199:11–122.
5. Hayes JM, Hann I, Punch LJ. The Bullet Related Injury Clinic-Healing the Deep Wounds of Gun Violence. JAMA Surg 2022;157(2):167–8.
6. Hansen LO, Tinney B, Asomugha CN, et al. "You get caught up": youth decision-making and violence. J Prim Prev 2014;35(1):21–31.
7. Monopoli WJ, Myers RK, Paskewich BS, et al. Generating a core set of outcomes for hospital-based violence intervention programs. J Interpers Violence 2021; 36(9–10):4771–86.
8. Gorman E, Coles Z, Baker N, et al. Beyond recidivism: hospital-based violence intervention and early health and social outcomes. J Am Coll Surg 2022. https://doi.org/10.1097/XCS.0000000000000409.
9. Corbin TJ, Rich JA, Bloom SL, et al. Developing a trauma-informed, emergency department-based intervention for victims of urban violence. J Trauma & Dissociation 2011;12(5):510–25. https://doi.org/10.1080/15299732.2011.593260.
10. Purtle J, Carter PM, Cunningham R, et al. Treating youth violence in hospital and emergency department settings. Adolesc Med State Art Rev. Fall 2016;27(2): 351–63.
11. Pino EC, Fontin F, Dugan E. Chapter 11: Violence intervention advocacy program and community interventions. In: Lee LK, Fleegler EW, editors. *Pediatric Firearm Injuries and Fatalities: The Clinician's Guide to Policies and Approaches to Firearm Harm Prevention.* 1st Ed. Springer Cham; 2021. p. 157–77.
12. Zun LSDL, Rosen J. The effectiveness of an ED-based violence prevention program. Am J Emerg Med 2006;24(1):8–13.
13. Cooper CED, Stolley PD. Hospital-based violence intervention programs work. J Trauma 2006;61(3):534–7.
14. Juillard CCL, Allen I, Pirracchio R, et al. A decade of hospital-based violence intervention: benefits and shortcomings. J Trauma Acute Care Surg 2016 2016; 81(6):1156–61.
15. Myers RK, Vega L, Culyba AJ, et al. The psychosocial needs of adolescent males following interpersonal assault. J Adolesc Health 2017;61(2):262–5. https://doi.org/10.1016/j.jadohealth.2017.02.022.
16. Butts JA, Roman CG, Bostwick L, et al. Cure violence: a public health model to reduce gun violence. Annu Rev Public Health 2015;36:39–53. https://doi.org/10.1146/annurev-publhealth-031914-122509.
17. Webster DW, Whitehill JM, Vernick JS, et al. Effects of Baltimore's safe streets program on gun violence: a replication of Chicago's ceasefire program. J Urban Health 2012;90(1):27–40.

18. Hureau DM, Wilson T, Rivera-Cuadrado W, et al. The experience of secondary traumatic stress among community violence interventionists in Chicago. Prev Med 2022;165(Pt A):107186.

19. MacGillis A. Can Community Programs Help Slow the Rise in Violence? ProPublica. Available at: https://www.propublica.org/article/are-community-violence-interruption-programs-effective. Accessed March 8, 2023.

20. How does public health tackle gun violence? Gun violence. Available at: https://www.apha.org/topics-and-issues/gun-violence. Accessed May 7, 2023.

21. Braga AA, Weisburd DL. Focused deterrence and the prevention of violent gun injuries: practice, theoretical principles, and scientific evidence. Annu Rev Public Health 2015;36:55–68.

22. Sierra-Arevalo M, Charette Y, Papachristos AV. Evaluating the effect of project longevity on group-involved shootings and homicides in New Haven, Connecticut. Crime Delinquen 2017;63(4):446–67.

23. Fischer KR, Bakes KM, Corbin TJ, et al. Trauma-informed care for violently injured patients in the emergency department. Ann Emerg Med 2019;73(2):193–202.

24. Hawkins BE, Coupet E Jr, Saint-Hilaire S, et al. Trauma-informed acute care of patients with violence-related injury. J Interpers Violence 2022;37(19–20):NP18376–93.

25. South ECMJ, Reina V. Association between structural housing repairs for low-income homeowners and neighborhood crime. JAMA Netw Open 2021;4(7). https://doi.org/10.1001/jamanetworkopen.2021.17067.

26. Heinze JE, Krusky-Morey A, Vagi KJ, et al. Busy streets theory: the effects of community-engaged greening on violence. Am J Community Psychol 2018;62(1–2):101–9.

27. Moyer RMJ, Ridgeway G, Branas CC. Effect of remediating blighted vacant land on shootings: a citywide cluster randomized trial. Am J Public Health 2019;109(1):140–4.

28. Gong CH, Bushman G, Hohl BC, et al. Community engagement, greening, and violent crime: a test of the greening hypothesis and Busy Streets. Am J Community Psychol 2023;71(1–2):198–210.

29. Richardson M-A. Framing community-based interventions for gun violence: a review of the literature. Health Soc Work 2019;44(4):259–70.

30. Engel RS, Corsaro N, Tillyer MS. Evaluation of the Cincinnati initiative to reduce violence (CIRV). Cincinnati, OH: University of Cincinnati Policing Institute; 2010. p. 354.

31. Cherpitel CJ, Ye Y, Bond J, et al. Alcohol attributable fraction for injury morbidity from the dose-response relationship of acute alcohol consumption: emergency department data from 18 countries. Addiction 2015;110(11):1724–32.

32. Hohl BC, Wiley S, Wiebe DJ, et al. Association of drug and alcohol use with adolescent firearm homicide at individual, family, and neighborhood levels. JAMA Intern Med 2017;177(3):317–24.

33. Boles SM, Miotto K. Substance and violence: A review of the literature. Aggression and Violent Behavior 2003;8(2):155–74.

34. Fagan J. Interactions among drugs, alcohol, and violence. Health Aff 1993;12(4):65–79.

35. Bell TM, Gilyan D, Moore BA, et al. Long-term evaluation of a hospital-based violence intervention program using a regional health information exchange. J Trauma Acute Care Surg 2018;84(1):175–82.

36. Cunningham RM, Carter PM, Ranney M, et al. Violent reinjury and mortality among youth seeking emergency department care for assault-related injury: a 2-year prospective cohort study. JAMA Pediatr 2015;169(1):63–70.
37. Pino EC, Fontin F, James TL, et al. Boston violence intervention advocacy program: challenges and opportunities for client engagement and goal achievement. Acad Emerg Med 2021;28(3):281–91.
38. Coupet E Jr, Dodington J, Brackett A, et al. United States emergency department screening for drug use among assault-injured individuals: a systematic review. West J Emerg Med 2022;23(4):443.
39. Carter PM, Cranford JA, Buu A, et al. Daily patterns of substance use and violence among a high-risk urban emerging adult sample: results from the Flint Youth Injury Study. Addict Behav 2020;101:106–27.
40. Goldstein PJ. The drugs/violence nexus: a tripartite conceptual framework. J Drug Issues 1985;15(4):493–506.
41. Jessor R. Problem-behavior theory, psychosocial development, and adolescent problem drinking. Br J Addict 1987;82(4):331–42.
42. Dicker RA, Thomas A, Bulger EM, et al, ISAVE Workgroup; Members of the ISAVE Workgroup. Strategies for trauma centers to address the root causes of violence: recommendations from the Improving Social Determinants to Attenuate Violence (ISAVE) workgroup of the American College of Surgeons committee on trauma. J Am Coll Surg 2021;233(3):471–8.e1.
43. Lee LK, Fleegler EW, Goyal MK, et al. Firearm-Related Injuries and Deaths in Children and Youth. Pediatrics 2022. https://doi.org/10.1542/peds.2022-060071.

Suicide Prevention in Pediatric Health Care Settings

Jeremy Esposito, MD, MSEd[a,b,c],*, Molly Davis, PhD[c,d,e,f],
Rhonda C. Boyd, PhD[c,d,e]

KEYWORDS

- Suicide • Prevention • Pediatric • Youth

KEY POINTS

- Suicidal thoughts and behaviors are prevalent among youth.
- Research has highlighted disparities in suicide risk.
- Evidence-based practices for suicide screening, assessment, and brief intervention exist, but there are barriers to implementing these practices in health care settings.

INTRODUCTION
Definitions

Suicide is a major public health problem. There are a range of actions that encompass suicidal ideation and behaviors, and it is important for clinicians to understand these differences when assessing patients (**Table 1**). For example, for suicidal ideation with a plan, a youth may have a thought to run into the street and get hit by a car to die while another youth may have a thought to access the household firearm to kill himself or herself. Suicide intent can be challenging to determine with younger children; thus a provider must rely on the child's thoughts and behaviors.[4] An example of an interrupted suicide attempt may be a youth having a plastic bag in their hand in his or her room

---

[a] Division of Pediatric Emergency Medicine, Children's Hospital of Philadelphia, 3401 Civic Center Boulevard, Philadelphia, PA 19104, USA; [b] Department of Pediatrics, Perelman School of Medicine, University of Pennsylvania, 3400 Civic Center Boulevard, Philadelphia, PA 19104, USA; [c] Department of Psychiatry, Perelman School of Medicine, University of Pennsylvania, 3400 Civic Center Boulevard, Philadelphia, PA 19104, USA; [d] Department of Child and Adolescent Psychiatry and Behavioral Sciences, Children's Hospital of Philadelphia, 3440 Market Street, Suite 200, Philadelphia, PA 19104, USA; [e] Department of PolicyLab, Children's Hospital of Philadelphia, 3401 Civic Center Boulevard, Philadelphia, PA 19104, USA; [f] Penn Implementation Science Center at the Leonard Davis Institute of Health Economics (PISCE@LDI), University of Pennsylvania, 3641 Locust Walk, Philadelphia, PA 19104, USA
* Corresponding author. Division of Emergency Medicine, Children's Hospital of Philadelphia, 3501 Civic Center Boulevard, CTRB 2nd Floor, Philadelphia, PA 19104.
E-mail address: espositoj1@chop.edu

Pediatr Clin N Am 70 (2023) 1115–1124
https://doi.org/10.1016/j.pcl.2023.06.008
0031-3955/23/© 2023 Elsevier Inc. All rights reserved.

Table 1
Definitions for suicidal ideation and behaviors

Suicidal Ideation and Behaviors	Definitions
Suicidal ideation	Thoughts of harming or killing oneself, includes a range of wishes of death to suicidal ideation with intent and plan[1-3]
Suicide intent	How likely someone is to act on their suicidal thoughts[4]
Suicide attempt	Potentially fatal, self-inflicted destructive behavior with the explicit or inferred intent to die, can be interrupted by some outside circumstances, or the youth can stop the attempt himself or herself[1,2,5]
Suicide	Fatal, self-inflicted destructive behavior with explicit or inferred intent to die[1,2]

to put over his or her head and his or her parent coming into the room. For another youth, this may be running the car in the garage and a friend calling him or her on the cell phone, and he or she stops the attempt. Also included in a suicide attempt is preparatory behavior toward imminently making a suicide attempt. This can include writing a suicide note or giving things away, or gathering a specific method, such as collecting pills or a rope.

The language used to discuss and impart information about suicide risk has changed over time. There have been efforts to eliminate words and phrases that are offensive, imprecise, or biased. Words recommended for removal from suicide nomenclature include completed suicide, nonfatal suicide, failed attempt, successful suicide, suicidality, suicide gesture, manipulative act, and suicide threat.[6] In addition, it is important to avoid saying committed suicide as that term indicates suicide is a sin or a crime and reinforces stigma. It is preferable to state died by suicide.[7]

Current Trends

Suicide is the second leading cause of death for young people ages 10 to 24 years of age.[8] A study examining suicide deaths among 5- to 24-year-olds in the first 10 months of the coronavirus disease 2019 (COVID-19) pandemic in 2020 showed an excess of 212 suicide deaths associated with the pandemic.[9] Furthermore, groups that had higher suicide deaths than expected were males, 5- to 12-year-olds, 18- to 24-year-olds, non-Hispanic American Indian/Alaskan Native (AI/AN) youth, and non-Hispanic Black youth. Another study of 10- to 17-year-old youth who died by suicide in 2020 and 2021 demonstrated 990 deaths, with an average age of 14.9 years and the majority being non-Hispanic White and male.[10]

Research on youth suicide is growing. According to National Survey on Drug Use and Health, which is a survey of US households, among adolescents aged 12 to 17 in 2020, 12.0%, had serious thoughts of suicide; 5.3% made a suicide plan, and 2.5% attempted suicide within a year.[11] Data from the Adolescent Behaviors and Experiences Survey, which was conducted during January to June 2021 to assess student behaviors and experiences during the COVID-19 pandemic, showed that 19.9% of students had seriously considered attempting suicide, and 9.0% made a suicide attempt in the 12 months prior to the survey.[12] Using the nationally representative sample of high school students, the Youth Risk Behavior Survey (YRBS) demonstrated significant increases from 2011 to 2021 for serious thoughts of suicide, suicide plan, and suicide attempts; however, suicide attempts with injury did not change in this time period.[13] These statistics and trends clearly highlight the high prevalence of suicide-related thoughts and behaviors.

There are notable other trends. Youth suicide rates increase with age and boys are more likely to die by suicide than girls.[14] However, suicidal ideation and attempts are higher among girls than boys.[12] In the YRBS, the percentage of girls who seriously considered attempting suicide, made a suicide plan, and attempted suicide increased from 2011 to 2021.[13] Current research is showing that firearms are the most frequent mechanism of suicide, with hanging and poisoning being also widely used.[9,10]

There are health disparities in suicidal ideation and behaviors. Recent research has highlighted trends among youth of color that warrant attention. For example, a study of suicide deaths among Black youth (ages 5–17 years) highlighted a significant trend of increasing deaths for boys (2.8%) and girls (6.6%) from 2003 to 2017.[15] Similarly, AI/AN youths ages 5 to 24 years were also identified as a group whose suicide death rates increased during 2020.[9] The YRBS recent data from 2011 to 2021 found a few trends:

Black, Latino, and White students who seriously considered attempting suicide and made a suicide plan increased.

Black and White students who attempted suicide increased.

Asian students who attempted suicide decreased.[13]

Finally, LGBTQ (lesbian, gay, transgender, bisexual, questioning) youths have been identified as a high-risk group for suicidal ideation and behavior. The Trevor Project's national survey on LGBTQ youth showed that 45% of LGBTQ seriously considered suicide in the past year, and that rate was more than 50% for transgender and nonbinary youth specifically.[16] Recent YRBS data also demonstrated that LGBTQ students and students who had any same-sex partners were more likely than their peers to attempt suicide.[13] Increased awareness and understanding of the prevalence rates and trends of suicidal ideation and behaviors for youth of color and LGTBQ youth are needed so that appropriate screening and interventions can be implemented.

SUICIDE SCREENING, ASSESSMENT, AND INTERVENTIONS

Evidence-based practices for suicide prevention, including screening, assessment, and brief intervention,[17–19] have been developed and deployed across various health care settings.[20,21]

Suicide Screening Tools

Suicide screening for youth has been conducted in several settings, including emergency departments (EDs), primary care, and schools. There are publicly available tools that screen for suicide risk.[17,22] For example, the Ask-Suicide Screening Questions (ASQ) tool has been validated and used in various medical settings, such as EDs,[17] inpatient medical and surgical units,[23] and outpatient specialty and primary care clinics.[24] In primary care, depression screeners such as versions of the Patient Health Questionnaire (PHQ) that include questions around suicidal ideation have been administered,[25–27] in accordance with guidelines recommending universal adolescent depression screening in this setting beginning at age 12.[28,29] By default, as with the PHQ, adherence to these depression screening guidelines often results in suicide screening, given that suicide risk questions are embedded within many depression screeners. Additionally, some settings have implemented both a depression screener that incorporates questions about suicidal thoughts and behaviors and a suicide-specific screener to further gauge risk.[30] Importantly, depression screening does not detect all youth at risk for suicide who would be considered at risk on a suicide-specific screener.[31]

Unlike adolescent depression screening guidelines, it should be noted that guidelines for screening adolescents for suicide risk have been more mixed.[29,32] For instance, whereas the US Preventive Services Task Force concluded that the evidence was insufficient to recommend routine screening for suicide risk in children and adolescents in primary care, the American Academy of Pediatrics (AAP) has recommended universal suicide screening for youth ages 12 and older in clinical settings.[32] The Joint Commission requires individuals age 12 and older who are being evaluated or treated for a behavioral health condition as their primary reason for care to be screened for suicidal ideation using a validated tool. Further research examining the effectiveness of suicide screening for promoting risk identification and follow-up across pediatric health care settings, including more research involving suicide-specific tools, will be important for helping to guide best practices for youth suicide screening implementation.

Brief Assessment and Interventions

Following a positive suicide screen, a brief suicide safety assessment is typically recommended to better understand risk and inform follow-up care, unless the patient is clearly at imminent risk based on his or her screening and needs an emergency evaluation.[32] Commonly used, evidence-based suicide assessment tools include measures such as the Columbia Suicide Severity Rating Scale (C-SSRS) and the Suicide Assessment Five-Step Evaluation and Triage (SAFE-T).[18,33] A suicide assessment involves querying about suicidal ideation and behaviors, as well as protective factors such as reasons for living. By assessing risk and protective factors, the clinician can then determine next steps, such as whether to send the patient home or to emergency or crisis services. Trainings in suicide assessment tools are available online.[34]

Recent meta-analytic findings of studies involving youth and adults demonstrated that brief suicide prevention interventions were associated with lower odds of subsequent suicide attempts and increased likelihood of linkages to follow-up care.[35] Brief suicide prevention interventions mentioned in the meta-analysis included brief contact interventions (eg, telephone calls, letters, and postcards), care coordination (ie, bidirectional communication between the referring clinical team and the mental health care team receiving the referral), safety planning interventions, and other brief interventions (eg, therapies focused on problem-solving skills, techniques informed by motivational interviewing). The Safety Planning Intervention (SPI) is a commonly used brief intervention for addressing suicide risk.[19] The SPI includes several components:

Recognizing warning signs
Using internal coping strategies
Engaging in social settings and with specific people who can serve as a distraction
Reaching out to family or friends for help with the crisis
Contacting mental health professionals or agencies
Lethal means restriction (ie, making the environment safe)

The SPI is often implemented with adolescents and adults and was recently adapted to be a dyadic/triadic intervention for youths ages 6 to 12 and their caregivers.[36] Importantly, the SPI should be distinguished from no-suicide contracts (ie, an agreement between a clinician and patient in which the patient agrees not to harm or kill himself or herself and/or to seek help when experiencing suicidal thoughts), as experts have spoken out against no-suicide contracts given the lack of empirical support for their effectiveness in clinical settings.[37]

There is limited research concerning whether these interventions are effective with racially/ethnically diverse youth. For example, a care coordination intervention conducted in pediatric EDs was not as effective in linking youth of color with follow-up mental health care as with white youth.[38]

ADDRESSING BARRIERS

There are long-standing barriers for pediatric providers, patients, and families around identifying and managing concerns for suicide. Although there has been progress in recent years, there is a long way to go in order to overcome challenges faced across pediatric clinical settings and as a nation. Some barriers include mental health stigma, limited mental health specialists, a lack of linguistically and culturally concordant mental health providers, long wait times for evidence-based services, poor follow-up systems, lack of transportation, insurance and cost difficulties, and limited behavioral health training for general pediatricians and medical subspecialists.[39,40] One study found that for primary care settings, time constraints and competing demands were consistent barriers among clinicians and leaders, while those in specialty mental health settings reported challenges with coordinating services with schools and other community providers.[41] Additionally, many similarities in barriers were noted across evidence-based practices for suicide prevention (ie, screening, assessment, and brief intervention) and across settings (ie, primary care and specialty mental health).[41]

Local mental health services and pediatric settings will vary, but there are common steps and standards of care that can be implemented to address barriers and avoid disparities. In recent years, resources have been developed by experts to help pediatric providers integrate behavioral health practices into patient care. For example, the AAP published a mental health toolkit for pediatricians in 2021 that includes several resources to prepare practices to integrate suicide screening, assessment, and brief interventions.[42] Organizations such as Zero Suicide Institute, American Foundation for Suicide Prevention (AFSP), and Suicide Prevention Resource Center provide comprehensive guidance to improve suicide prevention and have resources to help if a patient or loved one dies by suicide.[43–45] One resource within the Zero Suicide Institute includes an organization self-study that can be used as an initial step for practices and health systems as they evaluate their current practices. Additionally, health care systems have implemented clinical pathways to help providers and minimize variability in care.[46]

A multidisciplinary approach is needed as pediatric clinical settings and health systems work to improve their current practices around suicide prevention. The AAP, AFSP, and National Institute of Mental Health recently created a Blueprint for Youth Suicide Prevention to help pediatric clinicians get started and advocate for change.[47] Each clinical setting, including pediatric hospitals, EDs, primary care sites, medical subspecialists, and pediatric behavioral health services, can identify suicide prevention champions to help gather resources, review the current care model, and plan for improved interventions. Input from a diverse team at the onset is ideal in order to get insight from all contributors, expedite solutions, and ensure diversity, equity, and inclusion. Pediatric clinicians, nurses, social workers, mental health providers, and patients and families with lived experience are examples of contributors to include in planning and monitoring practices. Other contributors could include quality improvement experts, as well as school and community members. A major overhaul of processes or initial interventions may take time. Pediatric clinicians are already under time constraints, and in order to incorporate the planning and training needed for effective change, protected time for frontline experts and other participants is essential. There are examples of successful integrated behavioral health initiatives when teams work together in clinical settings like primary care and the ED, especially when resources are provided and using quality improvement measures.[48,49] Each clinical setting can and must start somewhere.

CASE EXAMPLE

The following case is an example of integrating behavioral health care within clinical settings and communicating follow-up needs in the patient's medical home.

A 14-year-old boy with a past history of cardiac disease presents to ED with intermittent chest pain for 3 days. At triage, he seems to be in distress and is placed in a room. After initial evaluation and interventions, he is medically cleared. As part of the ED workflow, the ASQ is implemented and positive. The medical team talks to the patient alone, discusses concerns, and reviews the next steps. A behavioral health clinician assesses the patient, uses the C-SSRS, and determines that outpatient mental health services are appropriate. A safety plan is completed and lethal-means restriction is discussed prior to discharge. The ED communicates the suicide risk and follow-up recommendations to the patient's primary care provider, because it can be difficult for patients and families to access mental health care. The primary care site has integrated behavioral clinicians who reach out to the patient and family within 2 days after ED discharge to check in. The family reports being on a 4-month wait list for an outpatient mental health provider, and they make an appointment at the primary care site to bridge care until long-term behavioral health services are established. The primary care team is able to consult a psychiatrist via a telehealth visit to discuss medication management, and the patient visits the office every 2 weeks for symptom monitoring and brief, therapeutic interventions with a trained social worker until outpatient therapy is established.

SUMMARY AND FUTURE DIRECTIONS

With the growing personal and public health toll of youth suicide, it is essential that health care systems are prepared to address youth suicide risk across the various clinical settings where children and adolescents are likely to present. Fortunately, evidence-based practices for suicide screening, assessment, and brief intervention are available, and now focus should be on ways to partner with providers, health system leaders, patients, and families to determine optimal ways to consistently implement and sustain best practices for suicide prevention in health care settings. In particular, centering the voices of youth and families from historically marginalized backgrounds in the design and implementation of suicide prevention practices will be key for ultimately reducing health inequities. Integrated care models are a key avenue for fostering multidisciplinary collaboration around caring for youth with suicidal thoughts and behaviors.[48,49] Given limited resources (eg, staff) and time are commonly cited barriers to implementing evidence-based practices in health care settings,[50] looking for opportunities to task-shift and use digital mental health tools may be necessary for increasing the reach of suicide prevention efforts. Additionally, novel predictive modeling approaches for identifying suicide risk that utilize screening results and electronic health record data warrant further investigation.[51] Because several strategies are required to successfully implement suicide prevention practices in health care settings, yet those strategies are often under-reported in efficacy and effectiveness research, increases in transparent reporting about what it takes to implement suicide prevention practices will be critical for accelerating research-to-practice implementation.[52] The increased focus on youth mental health, particularly in the context of the COVID-19 pandemic, can pave the way for key prevention and intervention programming. Maintaining the momentum around these issues will be critical for saving young lives.

CLINICS CARE POINTS

- Suicide screening and assessment can be conducted in a variety of pediatric settings.
- There are resources for pediatric clinicians to prepare and build suicide prevention practices, such as the AAP Mental Health Toolkit.

DISCLOSURE

Preparation of this article was supported by the grants P50MH127511 (J. Esposito, R.C. Boyd) and P50MH115838 (M. Davis, R.C. Boyd). There are no other conflicts to disclose.

REFERENCES

1. Cash SJ, Bridge JA. Epidemiology of youth suicide and suicidal behavior. Curr Opin Pediatr 2009;21(5):613–9.
2. O'Carroll PW, Berman AL, Maris RW, et al. Beyond the Tower of Babel: a nomenclature for suicidology. Suicide Life Threat Behav 1996;26(3):237–52.
3. Bridge JA, Goldstein TR, Brent DA. Adolescent suicide and suicidal behavior. J Child Psychol Psychiatry 2006;47(3/4):372–94.
4. Crepeau-Hobson F. The psychological autopsy and determination of child suicides: a survey of medical examiners. Arch Suicide Res 2010;14:24–34.
5. Posner K, Brodsky B, Yershova K, et al. The classification of suicidal behavior. The Oxford handbook of suicide and self-injury 2014;8:7–22.
6. Crosby A, Ortega L, Melanson C. Self-directed violence: uniform definitions and recommended data elements (version 1.0). Atlanta (GA): Centers for Disease Control and Prevention; 2011.
7. Padmanathan P, Biddle L, Hall K, et al. Language use and suicide: an online cross-sectional survey. PLoS One 2019;14(6):e0217473.
8. Heron M. Deaths: leading causes for 2019. National vital statistics reports; vol 70 no 9. Hyattsville (MD): National Center for Health Statistics; 2021.
9. Bridge JA, Ruch DA, Sheftall AH, et al. Youth suicide during the first year of the COVID-19 pandemic. Pediatrics 2023;151. e2022058375.
10. Schnitzer PG, Dykstra H, Collier A. The COVID-19 pandemic and youth suicide: 2020-2021. Pediatrics 2023;151. e2022058716.
11. Substance Abuse and Mental Health Services Administration. Key substance use and mental health indicators in the United States: results from the 2020 national survey on Drug Use and health (HHS Publication No. PEP21-07-01-003, NSDUH Series H-56). Rockville, MD: Center for Behavioral Health Statistics and Quality, Substance Abuse and Mental Health Services Administration; 2021. Available at. https://www.samhsa.gov/data/.
12. Jones SE, Ethier KA, Hertz M, et al. Mental health, suicidality, and connectedness among high school students during the COVID-19 pandemic—Adolescent

Behaviors and Experiences Survey, United States, January–June 2021. MMWR supplements 2022;71(3):16–21.

13. Centers for Disease Control and Prevention. Youth Risk Behavior Survey. 2023. Available at https://www.cdc.gov/healthyyouth/data/yrbs/pdf/yrbs_data-summary-trends_report2023_508.pdf. Accessed March 15, 2023.

14. Ruch DA, Bridge JA. Epidemiology of suicide and suicidal behavior in youth. In: Ackerman JP, Horowitz M, editors. Youth suicide prevention and intervention. SpringerBriefs in Psychology. Cham: Springer; 2022. https://doi.org/10.1007/978-3-031-06127-1_1.

15. Sheftall AH, Vakil F, Ruch DA, et al. Black youth suicide: investigation of current trends and precipitating circumstances. J Amer Acad Child Adolesc Psychiatry 2022;61(5):662–75.

16. The Trevor Project. 2022 national survey of LGBTQ mental health. 2022. Available at: file:///C:/Users/rboyd/OneDrive/Documents/Paper/Pedclinicviolenceissue/trevor01_2022survey_final.pdf. Accessed March 15, 2023.

17. Horowitz LM, Bridge JA, Teach SJ, et al. Ask Suicide-Screening Questions (ASQ): a brief instrument for the pediatric emergency department. Arch Pediatr Adolesc Med 2012;166(12):1170–6.

18. Posner K, Brown GK, Stanley B, et al. The Columbia–Suicide Severity Rating Scale: initial validity and internal consistency findings from three multisite studies with adolescents and adults. Am J Psychiatry 2011;168:1266–77.

19. Stanley B, Brown GK. Safety Planning Intervention: a brief intervention to mitigate suicide risk. Cogn Behav Pract 2012;19:256–64.

20. Ballard ED, Cwik M, Van Eck K, et al. Identification of at-risk youth by suicide screening in a pediatric emergency department. Prev Sci 2017;18(2):174–82.

21. Sisler SM, Schapiro NA, Nakaishi M, et al. Suicide assessment and treatment in pediatric primary care settings. J Child Adolesc Psychiatr Nurs 2020;33(4):187–200.

22. Osman A, Bagge CL, Gutierrez PM, et al. The Suicidal Behaviors Questionnaire-Revised (SBQ-R): validation with clinical and nonclinical samples. Assessment 2001;8(4):443–54.

23. Horowitz LM, Wharff EA, Mournet AM, et al. Validation and feasibility of the ASQ among pediatric medical and surgical inpatients. Hosp Pediatr 2020;10(9):750–7.

24. Aguinaldo LD, Sullivant S, Lanzillo EC, et al. Validation of the Ask Suicide-Screening Questions (ASQ) with youth in outpatient specialty and primary care clinics. Gen Hosp Psychiatry 2021;68:52–8.

25. Kroenke K, Spitzer RL, Williams JB. The PHQ-9: validity of a brief depression severity measure. J Gen Intern Med 2001;16:606–13.

26. Spitzer RL, Kroenke K, Williams JB. Validation and utility of a self-report version of PRIME-MD: the PHQ primary care study. JAMA 1999;282:1737–44.

27. Davis M, Jones JD, So A, et al. Adolescent depression screening in primary care: who is screened and who is at risk? J Affect Disord 2022;299:318–25.

28. Zuckerbrot RA, Cheung A, Jensen PS, et al. Guidelines for Adolescent Depression in Primary Care (GLAD-PC): Part I. Practice preparation, identification, assessment, and initial management. Pediatrics 2018;141:e20174081.

29. US Preventive Services Task Force. Screening for depression and suicide risk in children and adolescents: US Preventive Services Task Force recommendation statement. JAMA 2022;328(15):1534–42.

30. Kemper AR, Hostutler CA, Beck K, et al. Depression and suicide-risk screening results in pediatric primary care. Pediatrics 2021;148(1). e2021049999.

31. Horowitz LM, Mournet AM, Lanzillo E, et al. Screening pediatric medical patients for suicide risk: is depression screening enough? J Adolesc Health 2021;68: 1183–8.

32. American Academy of Pediatrics. Suicide: blueprint for youth suicide prevention. 2023. Available at: https://www.aap.org/en/patient-care/blueprint-for-youth-suicide-prevention/strategies-for-clinical-settings-for-youth-suicide-prevention/conducting-a-brief-suicide-safety-assessment/. Accessed March 15, 2023.

33. Suicide Assessment Five-step Evaluation and Triage (SAFE-T) for Mental Health Professionals; 2009. Available at: http://www.mentalhealthscreening.org. Accessed March 15, 2023.

34. National Institute of Mental Health. Suicide risk screening training: how to manage patients at risk for suicide. 2019. Available at Suicide Risk Screening Training: how to manage patients at risk for suicide - YouTube. Available at: https://youtu.be/P4_-SF9lQuc. Accessed March 15, 2023.

35. Doupnik SK, Rudd B, Schmutte T, et al. Association of suicide prevention interventions with subsequent suicide attempts, linkage to follow-up care, and depression symptoms for acute care settings: a systematic review and meta-analysis. JAMA Psychiatr 2020;77(10):1021–30.

36. Itzhaky L, Stanley B. The Safety Planning Intervention for Children (C-SPI): rationale and case illustration. Cognitive and Behavioral Practice 2022.doi: 10.1016/j.cbpra.2022.10.001.

37. Rudd MD, Mandrusiak M, Joiner TE Jr. The case against no-suicide contracts: the commitment to treatment statement as a practice alternative. J Clin Psychol 2006; 62(2):243–51.

38. Grupp-Phelan J, Stevens J, Boyd S, et al. Effect of a motivational interviewing–based intervention on initiation of mental health treatment and mental health after an emergency department visit among suicidal adolescents: a randomized clinical trial. JAMA Netw Open 2019;2(12):e1917941.

39. Schnyder N, Panczak R, Groth N, et al. Association between mental health-related stigma and active help-seeking: systematic review and meta-analysis. Br J Psychiatry 2017;210(4):261–8.

40. Toure D, Kumar G, Walker C, et al. Barriers to pediatric mental healthcare access: qualitative insights from caregivers. J Soc Serv Res 2022;48(4):485–95.

41. Davis M, Siegel J, Becker-Haimes EM, et al. Identifying common and unique barriers and facilitators to implementing evidence-based practices for suicide prevention across primary care and specialty mental health settings. Arch Suicide Res 2021 Oct;15:1 23.

42. Earls MF, Foy JM, Green CM. Addressing Mental Health Concerns in Pediatrics: A Practical Resource Toolkit for Clinicians, 2nd Edition. American Academy of Pediatrics. Available at: https://shop.aap.org/mentalhealthtoolkit. Accessed March 15, 2023.

43. Zero Suicide. Available at: https://zerosuicide.edc.org/. Accessed March 15, 2023.

44. American Foundation for Suicide Prevention. Available at: https://afsp.org/. Accessed March 15, 2023.

45. Suicide Prevention Resource Center. Available at: https://www.sprc.org/. Accessed March 15, 2023.

46. Suicide Risk Assessment and Care Planning Pathway. Children's Hospital of Philadelphia, Philadelphia, Pennsylvania. Available at: https://www.chop.edu/clinical-pathway/suicide-risk-assessment-and-care-planning-clinical-pathway. Accessed March 15, 2023.

47. Suicide: blueprint for youth suicide prevention. American Academy of Pediatrics. Available at: https://www.aap.org/en/patient-care/blueprint-for-youth-suicide-prevention/. Accessed March 15, 2023.
48. Herbst RB, McClure JM, Ammerman RT, et al. Four innovations: a robust integrated behavioral health program in pediatric primary care. Fam Syst Health 2020;38(4):450–63.
49. Esposito J, Lavelle J, M'Farrej M, et al. Responding to a behavioral health crisis: applying a new care model in the emergency department. Pediatr Emerg Care 2022;38(3):e1147–50.
50. Davis M, Hoskins K, Phan M, et al. Screening adolescents for sensitive health topics in primary care: a scoping review. J Adolesc Health 2022;70(5):706–13.
51. Haroz EE, Kitchen C, Nestadt PS, et al. Comparing the predictive value of screening to the use of electronic health record data for detecting future suicidal thoughts and behavior in an urban pediatric emergency department: a preliminary analysis. Suicide Life Threat Behav 2021;51(6):1189–202.
52. Rudd BN, Davis M, Doupnik S, et al. Implementation strategies used and reported in brief suicide prevention intervention studies. JAMA Psychiatr 2022; 79(8):829–31.

Firearm Injury Prevention

Kelsey A.B. Gastineau, MD[a],*, Sandra McKay, MD[b]

KEYWORDS

- Firearm safety • Gun safety • Unintentional firearm injuries • Safer storage

KEY POINTS

- Firearms are the leading cause of death for US youth, overtaking motor vehicle collisions in 2020. Approximately 65% are due to homicide, 30% are due to suicide, 3.5% are due to unintentional injuries, 2% are undetermined intent, and 0.5% are from legal interventions.
- In homes with firearms, the likelihood of unintentional death, suicide, and homicide is three to four times higher than those without firearms.
- Secure storage of firearms, having them locked, unloaded, and separate from ammunition, can prevent unintentional firearm injuries.
- Physician counseling combined with providing a locking device such as a cable lock increases the frequency of safer storage in the home.

 Video content accompanies this article at http://www.pediatric.theclinics.com.

INTRODUCTION

Firearms are the leading cause of death for youth in the United States.[1] In 2020, there were nearly 4400 firearm-related deaths of youth under 19 years old, surpassing deaths due to heart disease, cancer, and asthma, combined.[2] For every child who dies by a firearm, at least three more are injured.[3] Youth who suffer firearm injuries have higher health care visits and costs compared with noninjured peers.[4,5] For children who witness or experience violence, they are more likely to suffer from substance abuse, anxiety, depression, school disruptions, and other negative health risks in adulthood.[6,7]

A comprehensive public health approach is needed to reduce pediatric firearm-related injuries with interventions at the individual, household, community, and policy levels. According to the updated American Academy of Pediatrics (AAP) Policy Statement "Firearm-Related Injuries and Deaths in Children and Youth: Injury Prevention

---

[a] Department of Pediatrics, Monroe Carell Jr Children's Hospital at Vanderbilt and Vanderbilt University Medical Center; [b] Department of Pediatrics, McGovern Medical School at the University of Texas Health Science Center at Houston, 6431 Fannin Street, JJL 480, Houston, TX 77030, USA
* Corresponding author. 2141 Blakemore Avenue, Nashville, TN 37212.
E-mail address: kelsey.gastineau@vumc.org

Pediatr Clin N Am 70 (2023) 1125–1142
https://doi.org/10.1016/j.pcl.2023.07.003
0031-3955/23/© 2023 Elsevier Inc. All rights reserved.
pediatric.theclinics.com

and Harm Reduction," a multifaceted approach to reducing injury should be under-taken, including interventions both in the clinical and community spaces. This includes a harm reduction approach toward anticipatory guidance regarding safe storage of home firearms, investments in hospital and community-based violence intervention programs, and regulations for firearms as consumer product. Pediatricians are an indispensable element in this effort. The authors discuss each of these protective layers, focusing on the pediatricians' role in preventing firearm-related injuries and death for youth by promoting firearm safety, including the removal or safe storage of firearms from places where children live and play.

EPIDEMIOLOGY

Unsecured firearms place children at risk for all types of firearm injury and death including unintentional injury, suicide, homicide, and mass violence such as school shootings. The United States has the highest rate of firearm-related injury and death in the world. The rate of firearm-related mortality in US youth was 36.5 times higher than other high-income countries in 2016 (4.02 per 100,000 vs 0.11 per 100,000).[8] Globally, approximately 90% of all firearm deaths in children aged 0 to 14 years occur in the United States.[9]

Using data from the Centers for Disease Control and Prevention (CDC), approximately 65% of pediatric (aged 0–19) firearm-related deaths in the United States are homicides, 30% are suicides, 3.5% are due to unintentional injuries, 2% are undetermined intent, and 0.5% are from legal interventions.[2] Note that the term "unintentional" is used opposed to "accident" throughout as the term accident refers to events that cannot be prevented and most unintentional firearm injuries are preventable.

Disparities in Firearm Injuries and Deaths

The burden of firearm-related injuries and deaths is not distributed equally, and differences exist by age, gender identity, region, and race and ethnicity (**Figs. 1** and **2**). Overall, older children, males, and populations made to be minoritized including Black and Hispanic youth are disproportionately affected. Of US youth who died of a firearm-related injury in 2020, males represented 86% and youth aged 15 to 19 years represented 78%.[2] Individuals in the Lesbian, Gay, Bisexual, Transexual, Queer community (LGBTQ+) are more than twice as likely to be victim of firearm injury than their cisgender and straight peers (11.5 vs 4.6 per 1000).[10] Although overall death rates from firearm injuries among youth are similar in rural and urban communities, differences exist by intent. Rates of firearm suicide are higher among youth from rural areas and urban youth have higher rates of firearm homicide.[11,12] Children in the South experience the highest rates of firearm-related injury and death with the South region accounting for half of all deaths of children aged 0 to 19 years in 2020.[13]

Significant racial disparities exist across firearm injury intents and have been widening in the last decade.[14] These disparities are not due to differences at a biologic or genetic level, but rather a result of historical and ongoing structural racism.[15] Violence disproportionately occurs in communities experiencing economic and social inequities, including concentrated poverty, disinvestment, and residential racial segregation.[16] To advance health equity, we must also address the root causes contributing to systemic racism to truly impact firearm injury at all levels.

Unintentional Deaths

In 2020, there were 149 unintentional deaths in youth aged 0 to 19 years.[2] Although there was a downward trend from 2011 to 2015, unintentional firearm death rates

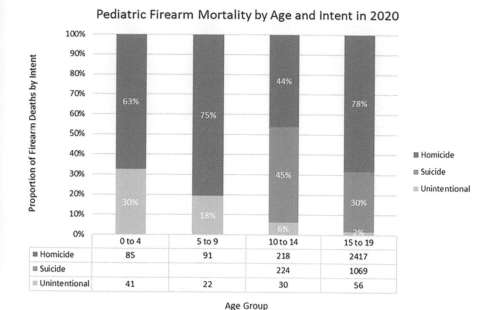

Fig. 1. Firearm mortality by age and intent. (Figure created with data from the overall firearm causes of injury related deaths from age 0 to 19 by intent from 2022, as compiled by National Center for Health Statistics. Suicide data only includes ages 10-19.)

have not substantially changed since 2011 (age-adjusted rate 0.18 per 100,000 in 2020 vs 0.17 per 100,000 in 2011).[2] Unintentional injuries occur more commonly in younger children compared with older age groups.[3] For children aged 0 to 4 years, unintentional injuries make up 30% of all compared with 18% for 5 to 9-year-olds, 6.1% for 10 to 14-year-olds, and 1.5% for 15 to 19-year-olds.[2] The case fatality rates for youth sustaining unintentional firearm injuries are lower (1%–6%), compared those sustaining injuries due to assault (19%) or self-inflicted injuries (85%).[3,17]

For younger children (aged 0–12 years), most firearm deaths (85%) from occur in the home.[3] The most common circumstance surrounding unintentional firearm deaths of both younger (60%) and older children (49%) was playing with a gun.[3]

When considering unintentional injuries, it is important to examine outcomes when children access unauthorized firearms. Findings from Everytown's #NotAnAccident Index show that there were at least 2070 unintentional shootings by children under 18 years old between 2015 and 2020, resulting in 765 deaths and 1366 injuries. Victims of the shootings by children were most often also children under 18 years. Furthermore, nearly 80% of shootings by children occurred in a home or car, and when the firearm type was known, handguns were involved in 85% of incidents.[18]

Suicide

There has been a rapid increase in the rate of firearm suicide among youth in the United States with 1293 youth aged 10 to 19 years dying by firearm suicide in 2020. In the past decade, there has been a 53% increase in the rate of firearm suicide among those 10 to 24 years old. For children aged 10 to 14 years, the rate of firearm suicide has increased by an alarming 146% during that same period.[2] The rate of non-firearm suicide increased by 25%.[2]

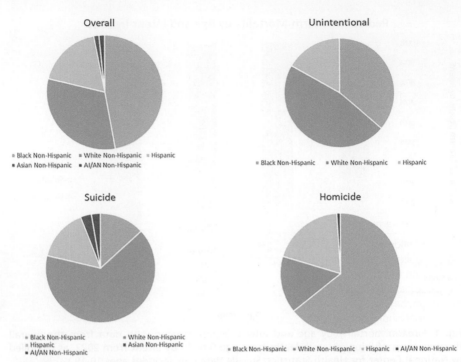

Fig. 2. Proportion of pediatric firearm mortality by intent and race/ethnicity. (Figure created with data from the overall firearm causes of injury related deaths from age 0 to 19 by intent from 2022, as compiled by National Center for Health Statistics. Suicide data only includes ages 10-19. Some categories had unstable values (<20 deaths) and are therefore not represented.)

Boys and young men are disproportionately affected by suicide, representing nearly 9 out of 10 suicide victims.[2] Young American Indian and Alaska Native youth have the highest rate of firearm suicide. Over the past decade, all racial groups have seen an increase in the rate of firearm suicide. Asian and Pacific Islanders historically have the lowest risk. However, this population has experienced the largest increase with the rate of firearm suicide in youth aged 10 to 19 years increasing by 150% in this group compared with 120% for Black youth, 100% for Hispanic youth, 88% for American Indian or Alaska Native, and 36% for White youth.[2]

Firearms are a uniquely lethal means. The case fatality for suicide is 90% when a firearm is used. Conversely, 4% of suicide attempts that do not use a firearm are fatal.[19] In completed suicides in 2020, adolescent males used a firearm 54% of the time and adolescent females used a firearm 22% of the time.[2] The mere presence of a firearm in the home increases the risk of adolescent suicide by fourfold.[20] In addition, more than a third of adolescents nationwide report that they can access a loaded firearm within five minutes.[21]

Homicide

Rates of firearm-related homicide have been increasing nearly every year since 2011, now 76% higher than a decade ago (age-adjusted rate 3.39 vs 1.93 per 100,000).[2] There were 2811 youth who died by firearm-related homicide in 2020, representing 136,528 years of potential life lost.[2]

In the context of homicide, younger children (0–12 years old) are more likely to be shot by an adult they know in situations of intimate partner violence or another crime.[3] Older children (13–17 years) are equally likely to be killed at home (39%) or on the street or sidewalk (38%).[3] Adolescents are more likely to be killed by a peer.[3]

Stark disparities exist when examining firearm-related homicides. In a recent study by Andrews and colleagues,[14] the investigators found that Black youth had a 4.3 times higher firearm mortality rate compared with White youth. Community gun violence, a form of interpersonal firearm-related assault that occurs between non-intimately related individuals, is highly concentrated among a small number of people and microplaces.[22,23] This form of violence disproportionately impacts Black and Hispanic individuals living in underserved communities as a result of place-based discrimination.[24,25]

Nonfatal Firearm Injuries

For every youth who dies from a firearm-related injury, many more are injured, with 24,777 children and adolescents sustaining a nonfatal firearm injury in 2020.[2] In addition, youth who survive the initial injury often face long-term medical and psychological problems with nearly 50% of children hospitalized with firearm-related injuries being discharged with a disability.[26]

Youth are harmed not only as direct victims, but through indirect exposure as well, and the extent of this toll is yet to be fully known. Every year, approximately 3 million children and teens are exposed to gun violence.[27] Siblings are harmed when their brother or sister is killed with a gun. School children and communities are stricken by grief and fear after a school shooting. The long-term psychological impact to children and communities are still being investigated.

SCOPE OF THE PROBLEM
Ownership and Storage Patterns

According to data from a nationally representative survey in 2021, four in ten adults living with children, and subsequently 30 million children, live in a home with a firearm in the United States.[28] In the context of the unprecedented rise in firearm sales temporally related to the coronavirus pandemic,[29] there were 7 million more children living in homes with firearms than in 2015. As a result, at least 4.6 million children live in a home with a firearm kept unlocked and loaded, placing them at risk for harm.

The United States has the highest rate of firearm ownership in the world, with nearly 400 million civilian-owned firearms (120 firearms per 100 residents).[30] Firearm ownership varies by state and region as shown in **Fig. 3**. Firearm ownership also varies across demographic groups with higher ownership reported by men, White adults, and those living in rural communities.[31] During the COVID-19 pandemic, it was estimated that there were 7.5 million new firearm purchasers with demographics shifting away from the traditional White male to more women and more people of color.[32,33]

Reasons for Ownership

Two-thirds of firearm owners own more than one firearm.[31] Regarding types of firearms owned, 72% of firearm owners own handguns, 62% own rifles, and 54% own shotguns. The most reported reason for owning a firearm is for personal protection. This belief has increased from 26% of Americans in 1999 to 67% in 2017.[35] It should be noted here that firearms are used for self-defense in less than 1% of crimes and

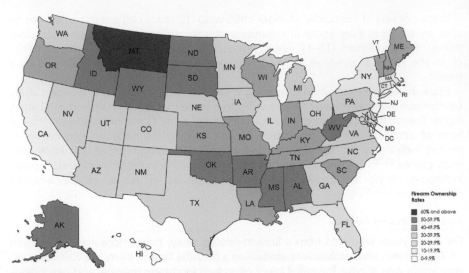

Fig. 3. State-level firearm ownership rates in the United States. (Data created from a 2020 RAND Corporation study "State-Level Estimates of Household Firearm Ownership."[34])

evidence shows that firearms in the home are associated with higher odds of firearm-related suicide, homicide, and unintentional injury.[36] Most firearm owners cite multiple reasons for firearm ownership and others include hunting (38%), sport shooting (30%), collecting (13%), and job requirement (8%).[31]

Risk of Unsecured Firearms

Access to a firearm in the home increases risk of harm given the natural curiosity and impulsivity of children. Access to a firearm in the home increases the risk for youth suicide, well summarized in a systematic review finding that access to firearms has a greater than three times pooled risk for completed suicide.[37] In incidents of gunfire on school grounds, 78% of shooters under the age of 18 years obtained the gun from their home or the home of a friend or relative.

Every year, 380,000 guns are stolen from private gun owners.[38] Many stolen firearms are then linked to crime, including 30% of firearms found at crime scenes as reported in a study from Pittsburgh, PA.[39] Based on a 2016 Survey of Prison Inmates, 90% of prisoners who possessed a gun during their offense did not obtain it from a retail source with 6% reported having stolen the firearm.[40]

During the pandemic, there were substantially limited opportunities for safety training, with many regions facing lockdowns and limits on in-person contact. Accordingly, the pandemic has led to a relatively new population of firearm owners who may not be as versed in firearm safe storage, highlighting the importance of developing effective education on firearm safe storage interventions.

Focus groups performed by Aitken and colleagues revealed that perception of injury risk to family members is overall very low, in which they are "more scared of snakes than of guns." There are also competing interests of the need for safe storage without delayed access for personal protection.[41] Recent surveys with Betz and colleagues[42] suggest that firearm owners prefer to choose their storage device via receiving a voucher or coupon. This suggests that parents can be educated but require access to a storage device of their choosing.

FIREARM SECURE STORAGE INTERVENTIONS

Storing firearms securely has a protective effect against firearm injury. *Secure storage of firearms is defined as having firearms stored locked, unloaded, and with ammunition locked and stored separately.*

Secure Storage

When firearms are securely stored, the risk of injury is reduced. In a case-control study, each specific practice of safe firearm storage including keeping a gun locked (OR 0.27), keeping a gun unloaded (OR 0.30), and storing ammunition locked (OR 0.39) and in a separate location (OR 0.45) was associated with a protective effect to reduce suicide and unintentional firearm injuries in homes with children and adolescents.[43] A recent modeling study estimated that up to 32% of youth firearm deaths by suicide or unintentional injury could have been prevented by securing household firearms.[44]

Firearm Secure Storage Options

There are a variety of options available for securely storing firearms when they are not in use. There are pros and cons to each outlined in **Table 1** and **Fig. 4**. The most appropriate device will depend on the family's reason for ownership and intended use of the firearm as well as the type of firearm(s) in the home. Storage devices can be purchased from gun retailers or sporting goods stores. Often local law enforcement agencies can provide free cable locks as a part of the national Project ChildSafe program, and many hospitals and community centers may have access to free cable locks.

Although removing firearms from the home is the most protective measure, this may not be the best situation for all families. If families are interested in removing firearms, options include storing the firearms with a trusted friend or relative, depending on the state laws, gun shops, shooting ranges, self-storage rental units, or local law enforcement.

It can be helpful to have some basic knowledge about firearms when providing secure storage counseling. There are two broad categories of firearms including short guns (pistols, handguns, and revolvers) and long guns (rifles and shot guns). Federal purchasing laws vary by state for long gun purchasing, but most individuals need to be anywhere between 18 and 21 years. Handgun purchases require one to be 21 years of age. Both short guns and long guns can be semiautomatic, which means that once it is fired, the cartridge is expelled and the next bullet is automatically loaded; however, it only fires one bullet at a time, as opposed to the fully automatic weapon which fires multiple bullets with the depression of the trigger. Several rifles require different actions such as a lever or pump action to load the next bullet so it can be ready to fire. Understanding the different types of firearms can be important when counseling families on what type of safety device may be best for their family.

In Video 1 (available online at http://www.pediatric.theclinics.com/), Dr Sandy McKay discusses general firearm safety principles and how common safety firearm devices are used.

Physician Counseling

Physician counseling during routine well-child examinations combined with the distribution of tangible tools for firearm storage is effective in increasing secure storage. Barkin and colleagues demonstrated in a large clinic-based randomized controlled trial that safe firearm storage behavior following a motivational interviewing program improved by 10%.[45] Providers can play a similar role in the hospital setting. Uspal and colleagues[46] reported that parents of children with mental health complaints

Table 1
Storage options for families

Method	Description and How it Works	Pros	Cons	Cost Range
Cable Lock	Device that blocks the chamber to prevent a cartridge from being fired. Chamber locks are inserted in or through the magazine well or chamber or are inserted through the gun barrel and chamber to block a cartridge from moving into position.	• Widely available • Inexpensive • Renders the firearm inoperable	• Cable can be cut • Do not work for every firearm	Free $10–$50 $2/item if ordered in bulk
Trigger Lock	A two-piece lock that fits over the trigger guard A rigid cylinder fits behind the trigger so the trigger cannot be pulled. A push-button keypad, combination, or key opens the lock.	• Inexpensive • Widely available. • Quick access (keypad models)	• Not generally recommended given multiple drawbacks • Can still potentially fire the weapon • May break easily • May not prevent theft, as some locks may be removed later	$5–$35
Lock Box	Handgun is locked inside the box. Can be locked with key, keypad, or biometric.	• Quick access if the lock is push-button or digital • Can secure multiple firearms • Mobile	• Can be more expensive • Only for handguns	$25–$350
Full Size Gun Safe or Vault	Safe in a variety of sizes designed to store long guns, handguns, or other valuables.	• Can secure multiple firearms • Prevents against thefts • Protects from damage	• Can be more expensive • Heavy and difficult to move	$200–$2,500

Guide to Secure Gun Storage Devices

Secure gun storage can be a lifesaver. It can prevent theft and access by children, unauthorized users, and anyone who may pose a danger to themselves or others. The best device for you is the one that is most appropriate for the circumstances in your household.

Full-Size Gun Safe
Storage of multiple guns in one place. Biometric lock more secure than key or passcode.
$200–$2,000

✓ Prevents access by children
✓ Prevents access
  by unauthorized users
✓ Prevents theft (if secured to
  a structure in home)
✓ Enables fast access

Lock Box/Locker
Smaller and lighter than safe. Biometric lock more secure than key or passcode.
$25–$350

✓ Prevents access by children
✓ Prevents access
  by unauthorized users
✓ Provides secure vehicle storage
✓ Enables fast access

Console/Vehicle Gun Safe
For storage in a vehicle. Biometric lock more secure than key or passcode.
$50–$350

✓ Prevents access by children
✓ Prevents access
  by unauthorized users
✓ Prevents theft (if secured
  to a structure in car)
✓ Provides secure vehicle storage
✓ Enables fast access

Gun Case
For home or in-transit storage of one firearm. Uses external lock.
$10–$150

✓ Prevents access by children
✓ Prevents access by
  unauthorized users
✓ Enables fast access

Trigger Lock
Locks trigger of single weapon. Never use with loaded gun. May be dismantled with minimal tools and skills, so not as effective with older children and teens.
$10–$75

✓ Prevents use by small children
✓ Enables fast access

Cable Lock
Cable runs through action of single weapon to prevent firing. Ammunition must be removed for lock use. May be dismantled with minimal tools and skills, so not as effective with older children and teens.
$0ᵃ–$50

✓ Prevents use by small children
✓ Enables fast access

Fig. 4. Secure storage device options for families. ᵃOften provided free with firearm purchase. (*Courtesy of* BeSMARTforKids.org.)

modestly improved safe storage behavior from 21% to 31% following lethal means counseling by emergency medicine physicians and psychiatrists. Physician counseling regardless of performed in the clinic or hospital setting can be an effective mechanism to disseminate firearm safe storage information.

The AAP recommends that pediatricians incorporate questions about the presence and availability of firearms into their patient history taking.[47] Just like counseling on seatbelts, pool safety, or vaccines, conversations about firearm ownership and secure storage should also be judgment-free and collaborative. See Box 1 for helpful a few helpful counseling tips. It can be helpful to provide families with a handout (**Boxes 1 2**) and a free cable lock so they can learn more about safe storage and lock their firearms.

Anticipatory guidance should also include asking about firearms in the homes of relatives and friends where the child(ren) may visit. This can be an emotional or uncomfortable topic for caregivers. Providing them with example strategies and solutions

---

Box 1
Counseling tips

1. Approach the conversation in a nonjudgmental and collaborative manner.

2. Consider presumptive language to start the conversation. Then, follow-up with open-ended questions to learn more about reasons for firearm ownership and interest in secure storage as needed.
   a. Examples:
      i. "Tell me about how you store firearms in your home and vehicles."
      ii. "Many of the families I care for have firearms and I'd like to talk about options for storing firearms to help keep your kids safe."
      iii. Ask "If firearms are present where your child lives or plays, how are they stored?"

3. Contextualize the discussion.
   a. Contextualize firearm safe storage around injury prevention and focus preventing unauthorized access to keep the child safe.

4. Involve the patient and family in finding a solution.
   a. Explain the rationale for secure storage and provide the family with options (*Box*), allowing them to choose which may work best for their situation.

5. Reiterate hidden does not mean secure.
   a. If a family tells you they trust their young child to not find a hidden firearm, affirm good intentions with a child's instruction and also encourage safe storage.
   b. In addition, remind families about the risks of an unsecured firearm being at risk for theft.

6. Provide trauma-informed care and practice cultural humility.
   a. Recognizing that many children and teens may have witnessed violence, experienced bullying, or other forms of trauma such as gun violence, trauma-informed practices in the clinical setting are important to address disparities.
   b. Consider the social and structural factors, such as limited economic opportunity or under-resourced schools, which may be impacting your patient and family.

7. Be intentional with word choice.
   a. Speak about firearms in the plural. Firearm owners generally prefer the word "firearm," and most owners own more than one firearm.
   b. Use the phrase "die by" or "die of" suicide instead of "commit" suicide to not assign blame or criminality.
   c. See "Talking About 'Firearm Injury' and 'Gun Violence': Words Matter" by Betz and colleagues[48] for more tips.

---

may be helpful, for example, including it in a text message with other safety concerns, such as allergen exposure, pool access, or pets.

Breaking Through Barriers to Counseling

Most health care providers agree that discussing firearm safety is important and beneficial. However, a small minority of providers regularly counsel families on firearm safety. Barriers to counseling cited by clinicians have remained largely unchanged over the past 2 decades and include lack of time, perceived parent resentment, and inadequate training.[49,50(p2)]

Caregiver Perspective

Most parents (75%) believe that pediatricians should counsel about safe firearm storage. Furthermore, in a nationally representative sample, 62% of firearm owners believed that firearm discussions are appropriate when there is a child in the home and 75% of the time if they believed a gun in the home increases suicide risk.[51]

Box 2
Resources for patient education

- Secure Storage Education Handouts
  - AAP (https://www-healthychildren-org.proxy.library.vanderbilt.edu/English/safety-preven tion/at-home/Pages/Handguns-in-the-Home.aspx)
  - JAMA Peds (https://jamanetwork.com/journals/jamapediatrics/fullarticle/2214029)
  - University of Michigan Injury Prevention Center (https://injurycenter.umich.edu/wp-content/uploads/2018/10/firearm_safety_flyer_final_11-10-2017_dhaas.pdf)
  - Children's Hospital of Philadelphia Center for Violence Prevention (https://violence.chop.edu/research-and-programs/gun-safety)
- Secure Storage Options Handouts
  - BeSMART for Kids (besmartforkids.org/wp-content/uploads/2022/12/Be-SMART-Secure-Storage-Comparison-FINAL.pdf)
  - National Sports Shooting Foundation (https://projectchildsafe.org/wp-content/uploads/files/PCS_SafeStorage_19.pdf)
  - Project Child Safe (https://projectchildsafe.org/wp-content/uploads/2020/12/PCSDigi talBrochure2020.pdf)

It is also important to note that there are no legal barriers to clinicians counseling on firearm secure storage. Currently, no federal or state laws or regulations exist prohibiting physicians from screening or counseling patients about firearms.[52]

Education

According to the 2019 AAP Periodic Survey, only 32% of pediatricians report receiving adequate professional training in firearm injury prevention counseling.[50] A 2019 survey of pediatric trainees reported low counseling rates with the most requested interventions to improve anticipatory guidance being education on technical aspects of safe storage (85.7%) and specific counseling language (80.5%).[53]

There is opportunity for undergraduate and graduate medical education programs to integrate firearm injury prevention into the curriculum.[54] McKay and colleagues developed a 2-hour multimodal workshop with short videos, expert-led didacts, and role-playing scenarios. This approach found increases in comfort and counseling probability 6 months after the workshop.[55] Quality improvement projects are also valuable ways for trainees and faculty to improve their counseling confidence, skills, and efficiency.[56]

In response to a call for firearm counseling education, the AAP developed a training program called "Safer: Safe Storage Prevents Harm" offered for Maintenance of Certification Part 2 credit.[57] The training provides relevant firearm injury epidemiology, risk mitigation strategies, and showcases brief common counseling scenarios. See **Table 2** for this and other online training resources.

FIREARM INJURY PREVENTION BEYOND THE CLINICAL SETTING
Educational Campaigns

Several studies have shown that teaching children about firearm safety is not an effective way to reduce risk for firearm injury or death. Many children know the storage location of home firearms and there is often discordance between parent's perception of children's knowledge and their behavior.[58] In addition, children as young as 3 years old are strong enough to pull the trigger of a gun.

Instead, we must rely on adults to prevent child access to unsecured firearms through secure storage practices.

Table 2
Educational resources for clinicians

Title	Length	Notes	Patient Resources	Countinuing Medical Education Available
Safer: Safe Storage Prevents Harm (AAP)	45–60 min	Universal firearm secure storage counseling for youth	Yes	Yes
Counseling on Access to Lethal Means to Prevent Youth Suicide (AAP)	1.5–2 h	Suicide prevention	Yes	Yes
BulletPoints (California Firearm Violence Research Center at University of California, Davis)	Asynchronous	Firearm injury prevention for youth and adults	Yes	Yes
The Physician's Role in Promoting Firearm Safety (American Medical Association)	1 h	Universal firearm secure storage counseling for adults and youth	Yes	Yes

One program example is the BeSMART campaign. It is a national, apolitical, nonpartisan message designed to help parents and adults normalize conversations about gun safety to prevent child gun deaths and injuries. The acronym stands for *Secure* all guns in your home and vehicles, *Model* responsible behavior around guns, *Ask* about the presence of unsecured guns in other homes, *Recognize* the role of guns in suicide, and *Tell* your peers to be SMART. BeSMART volunteers are available to discuss the firearm safety message at community events as well as in the health care setting.[56,59] You can find more information at BeSMARTforkids.org.

Community Level

Secure storage of firearms can directly and indirectly reduce firearm injuries. The number of stolen firearms is rising and is an important source of community violence. A 2017 study found that gun owners who owned more than 6 guns, owned guns for protection, and stored guns unsafely had a higher risk for having a gun stolen.[60] The best way to prevent firearms from being lost or stolen is to secure them in homes and vehicles.

Neighborhood level interventions, such as building restoration or greening, the process of restoring the landscaping and appearance of a vacant lot by cleaning, mowing, and maintenance, have been shown to decrease community safety concerns and gun violence.[61] Community violence intervention programs focus on reducing firearm injuries by establishing relationships and providing support to individuals at high risk of violence. Several models for community violence intervention exist including street outreach, group violence intervention, and hospital-based violence intervention programs.

Policy Level

At a policy level, stronger firearm safety legislation is associated with lower rates of firearm-related pediatric mortality.[62] Child access prevention (CAP) laws impose a legal penalty on an adult who fails to secure a firearm and leaves it available for a minor to access. There are no federal CAP or safe storage laws, and state laws vary. The strongest of these laws, often termed "negligence" laws, impose criminal liability when a minor gains access of a negligently stored firearm. The weakest of the laws prohibit someone from directly providing a firearm to a minor. In a study examining pediatric (aged 0–14 years) firearm deaths from 1991 to 2016, more stringent "negligence" CAP laws were associated with a 13% reduction in all-intent firearm fatalities, a 15% reduction in firearm homicides, a 12% reduction in firearm suicides, and a 13% reduction in unintentional firearm fatalities, but less stringent "reckless" CAP laws did not show an association.[63]

Broader policies considering upstream factors and structural inequality such as expanded unemployment insurance, increased public spending, and improved college affordability are also important in reducing firearm-related injury and death in youth by addressing the root causes of violence.[64,65]

SUMMARY

Firearms are the leading cause of death for youth in the United States. Nearly 4400 children and teenagers died in 2020. This equates to approximately 6 youth a day representing one classroom full of youth every school week. Beyond death and injury, exposure to violence has long-standing negative mental and physical impacts for youth. This is a critical public health problem that will take a comprehensive, multifaceted approach with pediatricians playing a key role.

Firearm injuries and deaths disproportionately affect Black youth, particularly Black adolescent males, and this disparity has grown in recent years. An equitable public health approach must also consider the root causes of firearm injuries including concentrated poverty, under-funded schools, under-resourced public support, and lack of economic opportunity.

Increased access to firearms in the home raises the risk of unintentional and intentional firearm injuries and deaths for youth. Secure storage, keeping firearms locked, unloaded, and separate from ammunition reduce this risk. Clinicians should provide universal secure storage counseling at all well-child checks and additional lethal means counseling for higher risk youth. Pediatricians should engage in nonjudgmental and culturally appropriate conversations with families to help them make the best decision for their situation.

As pediatricians we are called to address firearm injuries within the clinical encounter, but we must move ourselves outside of the clinical walls and impact change on a broader level. We can be guided by Dr Abraham Jacobi, the father of American pediatrics, who in 1904 said "It is not enough, however, to work at an individual bedside in a hospital... He is a legitimate advisor to the judge and jury, and a seat for the physician in the republic is what the people have a right to demand." To reduce the burden of firearm injuries and death in US youth, interventions must occur at the individual, household, community, and policy levels addressing inequities at each level. Pediatricians all too often see the devastating impacts of firearms on their patients and communities and can be a driving force for change.

CLINICS CARE POINTS

- Firearm secure storage counseling is an evidence-based recommendation from the American Academy of Pediatrics to reduce firearm injuries.

- Pediatricians should develop their own personal system of secure storage screening and counseling, incorporating. Counseling should be nonjudgmental, contextualized around injury prevention, and collaborative with the family.

- Use tools such as the electronic health record to prompt your questioning as well as links for families within your anticipatory guidance handouts.

- Empower families to normalize the conversation about secure firearm storage and recommend asking about the presence of unsecured firearms in the other homes children and teens visit.

DISCLOSURE

The authors of this article received no external funding and have no financial conflicts of interest to disclose.

SUPPLEMENTARY DATA

Supplementary data related to this article can be found online at https://doi.org/10.1016/j.pcl.2023.07.003.

REFERENCES

1. Goldstick JE, Cunningham RM, Carter PM. Current causes of death in children and adolescents in the United States. N Engl J Med 2022. https://doi.org/10.1056/NEJMc2201761. NEJMc2201761.

2. Injury Data Visualization Tools | WISQARS | CDC. Published January 11, 2022. Available at: https://wisqars.cdc.gov/data/non-fatal/home. Accessed January 11, 2022.

3. Fowler KA, Dahlberg LL, Haileyesus T, et al. Childhood firearm injuries in the United States. Pediatrics 2017;140(1):e20163486.

4. Ranney ML, Herges C, Metcalfe L, et al. Increases in actual health care costs and claims after firearm injury. Ann Intern Med 2020;173(12):949–55.

5. Pulcini CD, Goyal MK, Hall M, et al. Nonfatal firearm injuries: utilization and expenditures for children pre- and postinjury. Acad Emerg Med 2021;28(8):840–7.

6. Ford JL, Browning CR. Effects of exposure to violence with a weapon during adolescence on adult hypertension. Ann Epidemiol 2014;24(3):193–8.

7. Thompson T, Massal CR. Experiences of violence, post-traumatic stress, academic achievement and behavior problems of Urban African-American children. Child Adolesc Soc Work J 2005;22(5–6):367–93.

8. Cunningham RM, Walton MA, Carter PM. The major causes of death in children and adolescents in the United States. N Engl J Med 2018;379(25):2468–75.

9. Grinshteyn E, Hemenway D. Violent death rates: the US compared with other high-income OECD countries, 2010. Am J Med 2016;129(3):266–73.

10. Flores AR, Langton L, Meyer IH, et al. Victimization rates and traits of sexual and gender minorities in the United States: Results from the National Crime Victimization Survey, 2017. Sci Adv 2020;6(40):eaba6910.

11. Fontanella CA, Hiance-Steelesmith DL, Phillips GS, et al. Widening rural-urban disparities in youth suicides, United States, 1996-2010. JAMA Pediatr 2015; 169(5):466–73.

12. Rees CA, Monuteaux MC, Steidley I, et al. Trends and disparities in firearm fatalities in the United States, 1990-2021. JAMA Netw Open 2022;5(11):e2244221.

13. Patel SJ, Badolato GM, Parikh K, et al. Regional differences in pediatric firearm-related emergency department visits and the association with firearm legislation. Pediatr Emerg Care 2021;37(11):e692.

14. Andrews AL, Killings X, Oddo ER, et al. Pediatric firearm injury mortality epidemiology. Pediatrics 2022;149(3). e2021052739.

15. Formica MK. An eye on disparities, health equity, and racism—the case of firearm injuries in Urban Youth in the United States and Globally. Pediatr Clin North Am 2021;68(2):389–99.

16. Benns M, Ruther M, Nash N, et al. The impact of historical racism on modern gun violence: Redlining in the city of Louisville, KY. Injury 2020;51(10):2192–8.

17. Kaufman EJ, Wiebe DJ, Xiong RA, et al. Epidemiologic trends in fatal and nonfatal firearm injuries in the US, 2009-2017. JAMA Intern Med 2021;181(2): 237–44.

18. Everytown for gun safety #NotAnAccident index. Everytown Research & Policy. Available at: https://everytownresearch.org/maps/notanaccident/. Accessed February 28, 2023.

19. Conner A, Azrael D, Miller M. Suicide case-fatality rates in the United States, 2007 to 2014: a nationwide population-based study. Ann Intern Med 2019;171(12): 885–95.

20. Brent DA. Firearms and adolescent suicide: a community case-control Study. Am J Dis Child 1993;147(10):1066.

21. Salhi C, Azrael D, Miller M. Parent and adolescent reports of adolescent access to household firearms in the United States. JAMA Netw Open 2021;4(3):e210989.

22. Braga AA, Papachristos AV, Hureau DM. The concentration and stability of gun violence at micro places in Boston, 1980–2008. J Quant Criminol 2010;26(1): 33–53.

23. Braga AA, Clarke RV. Explaining high-risk concentrations of crime in the city: social disorganization, crime opportunities, and important next steps. J Res Crime Delinquency 2014;51(4):480–98.
24. Beard JH, Morrison CN, Jacoby SF, et al. Quantifying disparities in urban firearm violence by race and place in Philadelphia, Pennsylvania: a cartographic study. Am J Public Health 2017;107(3):371–3.
25. Jacoby SF, Dong B, Beard J, et al. The enduring impact of historical and structural racism on urban violence in Philadelphia. Soc Sci Med 1982 2018;199: 87–95.
26. DiScala C, Sege R. Outcomes in children and young adults who are hospitalized for firearms-related injuries. Pediatrics 2004;113(5):1306–12.
27. Finkelhor D, Turner HA, Shattuck A, et al. Prevalence of childhood exposure to violence, crime, and abuse: results from the national survey of children's exposure to violence. JAMA Pediatr 2015;169(8):746–54.
28. Miller M, Azrael D. Firearm Storage in US Households With Children: Findings From the 2021 National Firearm Survey. JAMA Netw Open 2022;5(2):e2148823.
29. NICS Firearm Checks: Month/Year. Federal Bureau of Investigation. Available at: https://www.fbi.gov/file-repository/nics_firearm_checks_-_month_year.pdf/view. Accessed February 20, 2023.
30. Karp A. Estimating global civilian-held firearms numbers, Small Arms Survey, 2018, 3-4. Available at: https://www.smallarmssurvey.org/resource/estimating-global-civilian-held-firearms-numbers, Accessed February 28, 2023.
31. Parker K, Horowitz J, Ingielnik R, et al. America's complex relationship with guns. Pew Res Cent 2017;16–28.
32. Lyons VH, Haviland MJ, Azrael D, et al. Firearm purchasing and storage during the COVID-19 pandemic. Inj Prev 2020. https://doi.org/10.1136/injuryprev-2020-043872. injuryprev-2020-043872.
33. Miller M, Zhang W, Azrael D. Firearm purchasing during the COVID-19 pandemic: results from the 2021 national firearms survey. Ann Intern Med 2021;M21–3423. https://doi.org/10.7326/M21-3423.
34. Schell T, Peterson S, Vegetabile B, et al. State-level estimates of household firearm ownership. Santa Monica, CA: RAND Corporation; 2020. https://doi.org/ 10.7249/TL354.
35. Dimock M, Doherty C, ChristianL 1615 L. St, Suite 800. Why Own a Gun? Protection Is Now Top Reason. Pew Res Cent. Published online March 12, 2013. Available at: https://www.pewresearch.org/politics/2013/03/12/why-own-a-gun-protection-is-now-top-reason/. Accessed February 28, 2023.
36. Hemenway D, Solnick SJ. The epidemiology of self-defense gun use: evidence from the national crime victimization surveys 2007–2011. Prev Med 2015;79:22–7.
37. Anglemyer A, Horvath T, Rutherford G. The accessibility of firearms and risk for suicide and homicide victimization among household members: a systematic review and meta-analysis. Ann Intern Med 2014;160(2):101–10.
38. Langton L. Firearms Stolen during Household Burglaries and Other Property Crimes, 2005–2010. Washington, DC. U.S. Department of Justice, 2012. Available at: https://www.bjs.gov/content/pub/pdf/fshbopc0510.
39. Fabio A, Duell J, Creppage K, et al. Gaps continue in firearm surveillance: evidence from a large U.S. city Bureau of Police. Soc Med 2016;10(1):13–21.
40. Alper M and Glaze L. Source and Use of Firearms Involved in Crimes: Survey of Prison Inmates, 2016, Washington D.C. U.S. Department of Justice, 2019.
41. Aitken ME, Minster SD, Mullins SH, et al. Parents' perspectives on safe storage of firearms. J Community Health 2020;45(3):469–77.

42. Betz ME, Stanley IH, Buck-Atkinson J, et al. Firearm owners' preferences for locking devices: results of a national survey. Ann Intern Med 2023. https://doi.org/10.7326/M22-3113.

43. Grossman DC, Mueller BA, Riedy C, et al. Gun Storage Practices and Risk of Youth Suicide and Unintentional Firearm Injuries. JAMA 2005;293(6):707–14.

44. Monuteaux MC, Azrael D, Miller M. Association of increased safe household firearm storage with firearm suicide and unintentional death among US youths. JAMA Pediatr 2019;173(7):657.

45. Barkin SL, Finch SA, Ip EH, et al. Is office-based counseling about media use, timeouts, and firearm storage effective? Results from a cluster-randomized, controlled trial. Pediatrics 2008;122(1):e15–25.

46. Uspal NG, Jensen J, Sanchez-Erebia L, et al. Emergent mental health visits to a pediatric hospital: impact on firearm storage practices. Pediatr Emerg Care 2021; 37(12):e1382–7.

47. Hagan JF, Shaw JS, Duncan PM, editors. Bright Futures: Guidelines for Health Supervision of Infants, Children, and Adolescents. 4th edition. Elk Grove Village, IL: American Academy of Pediatrics; 2017.

48. Betz ME, Harkavy-Friedman J, Dreier FL, et al. Talking about "firearm injury" and "gun violence": words matter. Am J Public Health 2021;111(12):2105–10.

49. Cheng TL, DeWitt TG, Savageau JA, et al. Determinants of counseling in primary care pediatric practice: physician attitudes about time, money, and health issues. Arch Pediatr Adolesc Med 1999;153(6):629.

50. Trends over 25 Years in Pediatricians' Involvement in Gun Injury Prevention. Available at: http://www.aap.org/en/research/pas-abstracts/trends-over-25-years-in-pediatricians-involvement-in-gun-injury-prevention/. Accessed July 25, 2022.

51. Betz ME, Azrael D, Barber C, et al. Public opinion regarding whether speaking with patients about firearms is appropriate. Ann Intern Med 2016;165(8):543–50.

52. Wintemute GJ, Betz ME, Ranney ML. Yes, you can: physicians, patients, and firearms. Ann Intern Med 2016;165(3):205–13.

53. Hoops K, Crifasi C. Pediatric resident firearm-related anticipatory guidance: why are we still not talking about guns? Prev Med 2019;124:29–32.

54. Puttagunta R, Coverdale TR, Coverdale J. What is taught on firearm safety in undergraduate, graduate, and continuing medical education? A review of educational programs. Acad Psychiatry 2016;40(5):821–4.

55. McKay S, Bagg M, Patnaik A, et al. Addressing firearm safety counseling: integration of a multidisciplinary workshop in a pediatric residency program. J Grad Med Educ 2020;12(5):591–7.

56. Gastineau KAB, Stegall CL, Lowrey LK, et al. Improving the frequency and documentation of gun safety counseling in a resident primary care clinic. Acad Pediatr 2021;21(1):117–23.

57. Safer: Storing Firearms Prevents Harm - AAP. Available at: https://shop.aap.org/safer-storing-firearms-prevents-harm/. Accessed July 6, 2022.

58. Baxley F, Miller M. Parental misperceptions about children and firearms. Arch Pediatr Adolesc Med 2006;160(5):542.

59. Silver AH, Azzarone G, Dodson N, et al. A randomized controlled trial for parents of hospitalized children: keeping kids safe from guns. Hosp Pediatr 2021;11(7):691–702.

60. Hemenway D, Azrael D, Miller M. Whose guns are stolen? The epidemiology of Gun theft victims. Inj Epidemiol 2017;4(1):11.

61. Gong CH, Bushman G, Hohl BC, et al. Community engagement, greening, and violent crime: A test of the greening hypothesis and Busy Streets. *Am J Community Psychol*, 71, 2023, 198–210.
62. Parikh K, Silver A, Patel SJ, et al. Pediatric firearm-related injuries in the United States. Hosp Pediatr 2017;7(6):303–12.
63. Azad HA, Monuteaux MC, Rees CA, et al. Child access prevention firearm laws and firearm fatalities among children aged 0 to 14 years, 1991-2016. JAMA Pediatr 2020;174(5):463.
64. Kim D. Social determinants of health in relation to firearm-related homicides in the United States: a nationwide multilevel cross-sectional study. PLoS Med 2019; 16(12):e1002978. Brohi K.
65. Rowhani-Rahbar A, Quistberg DA, Morgan ER, et al. Income inequality and firearm homicide in the US: a county-level cohort study. Inj Prev 2019;25(Suppl 1):i25–30.

Child Maltreatment

Destiny G. Tolliver, MD, MHS[a,1], Yuan He, MD, MPH, MSHP[b,c,1],
Caroline J. Kistin, MD, MSc[d],*

KEYWORDS

- Child maltreatment • Abuse • Neglect • Prevention
- Patient-centered medical home • Racism • Disproportionality

KEY POINTS

- Child maltreatment has serious physical and psychological consequences.
- Racism and bias have resulted in disproportionalities in child maltreatment assessment, reporting, and response, as well as inequities in access to community supports and other protective factors.
- Effective maltreatment prevention is a public health priority. The patient- and family-centered medical home has unique potential as a locus for prevention services.

BACKGROUND

Child maltreatment, which includes physical abuse, sexual abuse, psychological abuse, and neglect, is associated with serious health consequences, many of them long term.[1–5] Although each state has its own legal definition, the federal Child Abuse Prevention and Treatment Act defines child maltreatment as an "act or failure to act on the part of a parent or caretaker which results in death, serious physical or emotional harm, sexual abuse or exploitation," or an "act or failure to act, which presents an imminent risk of serious harm."[6]

Young children are at the highest risk for experiencing maltreatment and for suffering significant developmental consequences as a result.[7] In addition to the injuries and posttraumatic stress that can occur as a direct result of abuse and neglect, child maltreatment is associated with poor physical, mental, and emotional health years later in adolescence and adulthood, which may present as symptoms of anxiety

[a] Department of Pediatrics, Boston Medical Center, Boston University Chobanian & Avedisian School of Medicine, 801 Albany Street, Boston, MA 02119, USA; [b] Division of General Pediatrics, Children's Hospital of Philadelphia, 4865 Market Street, Philadelphia, PA 19104, USA; [c] Department of Pediatrics, Perelman School of Medicine at the University of Pennsylvania, Philadelphia, PA 19104, USA; [d] Division of Health Services, Policy, and Practice, Hassenfeld Child Health and Innovation Institute, Brown University School of Public Health, 121 South Main Street, Providence, RI 02903, USA
[1] Co-first authors.
* Corresponding author.
E-mail address: caroline_kistin@brown.edu

Pediatr Clin N Am 70 (2023) 1143–1152
https://doi.org/10.1016/j.pcl.2023.06.013
0031-3955/23/© 2023 Elsevier Inc. All rights reserved.

and depression, problem substance use, and a high prevalence of chronic conditions such as hypertension.[1–5] Child maltreatment is also associated with poor educational outcomes, including high rates of absenteeism, truancy, suspension, expulsion, and dropout, with long-term social and economic consequences and an increased likelihood of involvement with the criminal legal system.[8–11] In addition, although the associations are complex, child maltreatment may be transmitted intergenerationally. Adults who experienced child maltreatment seem to be at higher risk for having children who experience maltreatment as well, particularly in the setting of poor parental mental health and social isolation.[12,13]

PREVALENCE

In 2021, the most recent year for which national child maltreatment data are available, approximately 600,000 children in the United States were determined to be victims of abuse or neglect and 1820 children died as a result of maltreatment.[14] More than 25% of all children who experienced maltreatment were younger than 2 years.[14] Neglect accounted for most maltreatment cases (76% of substantiated cases), followed by physical abuse (16%), sexual abuse (10%), and psychological abuse (6%).[14] Since 1992, the annual rates of substantiated physical and sexual child abuse have declined significantly, dropping by more than 60%, whereas the annual rates of neglect have decreased by a more modest 13% over the same time period.[15]

During the coronavirus disease 2019 (COVID-19) pandemic, children and families experienced multiple stressors, including COVID-related caregiver deaths, financial strain, school closures, and disruptions in social services.[16–19] To date, evaluations of the impact of the COVID-19 pandemic on child maltreatment are mixed, with different studies demonstrating increases, decreases, and no change in prevalence, depending on the outcomes and populations examined.[20,21] Nationally, the number of maltreatment reports to child protective services, substantiated cases of abuse and neglect, and foster care placements have been lower in 2020 and 2021, compared with 2019, but it remains uncertain whether this reflects a true decrease in maltreatment, changes in reporting and investigatory practices, or other factors.[14] Forthcoming data from 2022 and future years will help illuminate maltreatment trends during the acute pandemic and recovery periods.

RACISM, BIAS, AND DISPROPORTIONALITY

There is a history of racism and bias in the assessment, reporting, and response to suspected child maltreatment by both clinicians and governmental agencies, which has especially impacted indigenous and black families in the United States.[22–29] Both interpersonal racism, between individuals, and systemic racism, including historical and present-day policies, practices, and norms that result in inequitable outcomes, contribute to disparities and racial disproportionality in child maltreatment.[22,30]

Racial disproportionality in the child welfare system refers to the overrepresentation or underrepresentation of families of certain races and ethnicities, compared with the proportion of the general population. For example, whereas white children make up the largest total number of children in foster care, indigenous and black children are disproportionally affected by out-of-home placement. In 2021, indigenous children made up only 1% of all children in the United States but were placed in foster care at a rate of 2 times their proportion in the population, whereas black children made up 14% of children in the overall population but 22% of the foster care population (a rate of 1.6 times their proportion in the population).[31] Nationally, compared with white, Latino, and Asian children, indigenous and black children have a significantly higher cumulative risk of removal from the home before age 18 years.[25]

With regard to maltreatment assessment and reporting by clinicians, a retrospective study of young children hospitalized with skull or long-bone fractures found that, compared with white children, black and Latino children had more than 8 times the odds of having a skeletal survey performed for further workup of suspected physical abuse, even after controlling for likelihood of maltreatment, appropriateness of the skeletal survey, and insurance status, and had more than 4 times the odds of referral to child protective services, after controlling for likelihood of maltreatment and insurance status.[27] A multisite study of young children hospitalized with head injuries found that, compared with white children, children of other races and ethnicities were significantly more likely to undergo further evaluation for physical abuse and to be reported to child protective services for suspected abusive head injuries.[28] These disparities in evaluation and referral practices varied considerably by clinical site and were most pronounced among children who were determined to be at low risk for abusive injury.[28] Child neglect, which is defined more vaguely than physical abuse, may be even more susceptible to disparate assessment and referral practices.[23]

At the state agency and social service levels, once referred for evaluation of maltreatment, black families are more likely than white families to undergo full investigations for abuse and neglect, have the reports substantiated, and have children placed in foster care but are less likely to receive supportive services.[22–25] Although interpersonal racism and bias can influence decision making at different stages in maltreatment assessment, system-level policies, practices, and norms that drive inequities play a role in these disparities as well.[22,23]

Historically, both indigenous and black families in the United States have been the targets of systemic family separation practices, with children removed from their homes for forced assimilation in the case of residential Indian schools and for profit in the setting of slavery.[22–24] These separations, which often resulted in child death, have left a legacy of intergenerational trauma and loss within communities, which is compounded by present-day inequities. There are multiple examples of laws and policies that have directly contributed to racial disparities in poverty, which is highly correlated with involvement with the child welfare system.[22–24] These examples include the discriminatory housing policies of the Federal Housing Administration in the 1930s, the deliberate exclusion of predominantly black domestic and agricultural workers from social security benefits in the 1930s, and, at the state level, the exclusion of predominantly black single-parent households from Aid to Families with Dependent Children benefits in the 1950s and the 1960s.[22–24] Of these the last one not only exacerbated financial strain in affected families but also led to heightened surveillance of households by the state and increased removal of Black children from their homes.[22–24]

With this legacy of interpersonal and structural discrimination in mind, equity must be a priority at the individual, institutional, and societal levels for maltreatment interventions and initiatives aimed at supporting families and preventing child abuse and neglect. Expert recommendations include training individuals who work with families to recognize and address personal biases and racism and develop cultural humility, disaggregating maltreatment process and outcome data by race and ethnicity to evaluate for disproportionalities and opportunities for intervention, and examining and supporting policy solutions that may narrow, rather than widen, disparities in maltreatment by race and ethnicity, including economic and social supports to families to reduce the risk of poverty.[22,23,26]

THE ROLE OF THE CLINICIAN AND THE MEDICAL HOME

The patient- and family-centered medical home has unique potential as a locus for supportive child and family services and offers the advantages of longitudinal relationships between clinicians and families, nearly universal access to care, a focus on preventive services, and frequent routine visits during early childhood when children are most at risk for maltreatment. At every clinical encounter, clinicians have the opportunity to connect families to health care services, community resources, and other supports that have been shown to prevent maltreatment. In addition, clinicians should recognize and respond to concerns for maltreatment; provide supportive care and continuity of services to children who have experienced abuse or neglect; support biological, kinship, and foster caregivers in each of their unique roles in caring for children in foster care; and advocate for policies and practices that strengthen all families.

Assessment and Response

Health care workers, including frontline clinicians, are required by law to report suspected child maltreatment to state child protective service agencies or other authorities.[6,32] Research has shown, however, that there are multiple factors that influence clinicians' responses to presentations of potential maltreatment, with marked variability in reporting practices and decisions regarding whether or not to pursue further evaluation.[33–38] In addition to the influence of racism and bias discussed previously, clinicians frequently cite a lack of knowledge about legal mandates and reporting requirements, uncertainty about the likelihood of maltreatment in specific cases, and poor experiences with prior referrals to the child welfare system as major drivers of their clinical decision making.[33–39]

In an effort to improve clinician assessment and referral practices, and decrease both underreporting and overreporting of maltreatment, some health care institutions have introduced the use of clinical guidelines and decision support tools, particularly for the evaluation and workup of child physical injuries.[40] The American Academy of Pediatrics has similarly published policy statements and guidelines for clinicians, including recommendations for the workup of suspected physical abuse,[41,42] as well as the recognition, evaluation, and prevention of abusive head trauma[43] and maltreatment of children with disabilities.[44] Consultation with experienced practitioners, including child abuse pediatricians, social workers, or other members of multidisciplinary child protection teams, may help clinicians more accurately assess risk and guide further workup.

In cases of potential child neglect, clinicians may need support to distinguish between maltreatment by a caregiver and unmet child needs due to poverty or other circumstances.[23] Similar support may be useful when clinicians note general signs that a child is struggling, such as social withdrawal or school failure, and are unclear on whether or how to explore whether there may be a component of maltreatment. Some states have developed systems to help mandatory reporters identify whether or not there are safety concerns that require child welfare involvement, and many child welfare agencies now include an "alternative response" option intended to focus on services for families with unmet needs but low concern for maltreatment.[14] The City of Philadelphia has proposed expanding the free "Philly Families CAN SupportLine" to serve all families with children up to age 17 years in connecting with supportive community services and home visiting programs, without involving child protective services.[45] If successful, the initiative, supported by the Philadelphia Departments of Public Health and Health and Human Services may serve as a model for collaborative family support in other cities.

Supportive Care

In many cases, the medical home can provide important continuity of care for children impacted by maltreatment. Clinicians should aim to provide trauma-informed care, including establishing a safe and supportive clinical environment, and should recognize the many ways that trauma may present, both in children and their caregivers.[46] In addition to providing routine medical services and supporting child growth and development, clinicians should anticipate the need for collaboration with behavioral health services and increased care coordination, including communication with multiple caregivers and child welfare agencies.[7,47] Children who have experienced complex trauma may require clinician advocacy and guidance to access necessary accommodations and supports at school through individualized educational plans, as well as physical therapy, occupational therapy, and behavioral and emotional supports through programs such as Early Intervention and other publicly-funded services. Trauma-focused cognitive behavioral therapy, and other trauma-specific interventions, may be particularly helpful.

Prevention and Advocacy

Effective maltreatment prevention is a public health priority and should be a focus of clinicians who care for children.[48s] The American Academy of Pediatrics has specifically called on pediatricians to "provide helpful guidance and refer families to programs and other resources with the goal of strengthening families, preventing child maltreatment, and enhancing child development."[49] Clinicians can engage in prevention-focused work with individual families, within their institutions, and in the broader community through support and advocacy for effective, family-centered policies.

With individual families, clinicians can focus on protective factors associated with maltreatment prevention, including caregiver knowledge of child development and positive parenting practices that support child social and emotional well-being.[50] Clinicians should screen for material needs, such as food and housing insecurity, and help connect families to relevant clinic- and community-based resources that help address identified needs. Given the intricate link between child and caregiver health, clinicians should consider dyadic models of care or close collaboration with adult health care practitioners to ensure family members' health care needs are being met. In addition to screening for postpartum depression at the recommended 1-, 2-, 4-, and 6-month infant visits, clinicians should routinely ask caregivers about stressors and supports in place, with referrals to clinic- or community-based behavioral health resources as needed.

At the institutional level, clinicians can advocate for colocation of supportive resources, including food pantries and diaper banks, which help families meet their material needs and decrease household stress.[51,52] Cross-sector collaborations that integrate other services into the medical home may effectively address additional social determinants of health. Examples include medical-legal partnerships that facilitate free legal aid for housing and educational advocacy, medical-financial partnerships that help families unlock financial savings and tax credits, and childcare navigation supports.[53–55] Clinicians should examine institutional policies and advocate for changes that center families and decrease the likelihood of unnecessary referrals to child protective services. For instance, automatic maltreatment reporting for all infants with prenatal substance exposure, regardless of the parent's recovery status or engagement with clinical care, can lead to mistrust and disengagement with health care, further worsening disparities in care and child welfare involvement.[56]

In the community, there is ample evidence that factors such as access to safe, affordable housing are closely associated with a decreased risk of maltreatment reports.[57,58] Clinicians should advocate for neighborhood- and system-level supports for families and children, including quality housing, safe neighborhoods, healthy food, high-quality affordable childcare, and paid parental leave. There is evidence that systemic initiatives that provide cash payments, including the Earned Income Tax Credit (EITC) and Child Tax Credit may be particularly promising approaches to preventing maltreatment.[59–61] Receipt of state-level refundable EITC is associated with a decrease in hospital admissions for abusive head trauma in young children, and states that provide a higher dollar amount of refundable EITC benefits have fewer state-level reports of child neglect, compared with states with lower benefits.[59,60] As of the beginning of 2023, however, only 31 states and the District of Colombia offer a state EITC. Differences in geographic availability, along with federal and state eligibility restrictions, may widen instead of narrow disparities in maltreatment outcomes and should be examined further.

SUMMARY

Child maltreatment is associated with significant morbidity, and prevention is a public health priority. Given evidence of interpersonal and structural racism in child protective service assessment and response, equity must be prioritized for both acute interventions and preventive initiatives aimed at supporting children and their families. Clinicians who care for children are well-positioned to support families, and the patient-centered medical home, in collaboration with community-based services, has unique potential as a locus for maltreatment prevention services. Clinicians should advocate for policies that support families and decrease the risk of child maltreatment.

CLINICS CARE POINTS

- Clinicians should be familiar with the common presenting signs and symptoms of maltreatment, including injuries that are unusual for a child's age and developmental stage, and should consult practice guidelines and child abuse experts to help assess risk and guide further workup.

- Clinicians should be familiar with trauma-informed approaches to screening for and addressing child maltreatment, as well as community-based resources to support children who have experienced complex trauma.

- Individuals who work with children and families should understand the history of racism in child maltreatment and engage in training to recognize and address personal biases and develop cultural humility.

- Data regarding maltreatment processes and outcomes should be collected and disaggregated by race and ethnicity to evaluate for disproportionalities and identify opportunities for intervention and improvement.

- Prevention of child maltreatment should be a priority. Clinicians should screen for unmet material needs and refer families to resources; connect caregivers with medical care, including behavioral health supports; and advocate for policies like the EITC and Child Tax Credit that support families and children.

DISCLOSURE

The authors have no financial or other conflicts of interest to disclose.

REFERENCES

1. Irazuzta JE, McJunkin JE, Danadian K, et al. Outcome and cost of child abuse. Child Abuse and Neglect 1997;21(8):751–7.

2. Felitti VJ, Anda RF, Nordenberg D, et al. Relationship of childhood abuse and household dysfunction to many of the leading causes of death in adults. The Adverse Childhood Experiences (ACE) Study. Am J Prev Med 1998;14(4): 245–58.

3. English DJ. The extent and consequences of child maltreatment. Future Child 1998;8(1):39–53.

4. Hussey JM, Chang JJ, Kotch JB. Child maltreatment in the United States: prevalence, risk factors, and adolescent health consequences. Pediatrics 2006; 118(3):933–42.

5. Draper B, Pfaff JJ, Pirkis J, et al. Long-term effects of childhood abuse on the quality of life and health of older people: results from the Depression and Early Prevention of Suicide in General Practice Project. J Am Geriatr Soc 2008;56(2): 262–71.

6. S. 3817 — 111th Congress: CAPTA Reauthorization Act of 2010." www.GovTrack. us. 2010. February 22, 2023 Available at: https://www.govtrack.us/congress/bills/ 111/s3817. Accessed July 26, 2023.

7. Sege RD, Amaya-Jackson L. AMERICAN ACADEMY OF PEDIATRICS Committee on Child Abuse and Neglect Council on Foster Care, Adoption, and Kinship Care, AMERICAN ACADEMY OF CHILD AND ADOLESCENT PSYCHIATRY Committee on Child Maltreatment and Violence; NATIONAL CENTER FOR CHILD TRAUMATIC STRESS. Clinical Considerations Related to the Behavioral Manifestations of Child Maltreatment. Pediatrics 2017;139(4). https://doi.org/10.1542/peds. 2017-0100.

8. Leiter J, Johnsen MC. Child maltreatment and school performance. Am J Educ 1994;102(2):154–89.

9. Porche MV, Fortuna LR, Lin J, et al. Childhood trauma and psychiatric disorders as correlates of school dropout in a national sample of young adults. Child Dev 2011;82(3):982–98.

10. Romano E, Babchishin L, Marquis R, et al. Childhood Maltreatment and Educational Outcomes. Trauma Violence Abuse 2015;16(4):418–37.

11. Sinko L, He Y, Tolliver D. Recognizing the Role of Health Care Providers in Dismantling the Trauma-to-Prison Pipeline. Pediatrics 2021;147(5).

12. Berlin LJ, Appleyard K, Dodge KA. Intergenerational continuity in child maltreatment: mediating mechanisms and implications for prevention. Child Dev 2011; 82(1):162–76.

13. Assink M, Spruit A, Schuts M, et al. The intergenerational transmission of child maltreatment: A three-level meta-analysis. Child Abuse Negl 2018;84:131–45.

14. U.S. Department of Health & Human Services, Administration for Children and Families, Administration on Children, Youth and Families, Children's Bureau. (2023). Child Maltreatment 2021. Available at: https://www.acf.hhs.gov/cb/data-research/child-maltreatment. Accessed July 26, 2023.

15. Finkelhor D, Saito K, Jones L. Updated Trends in Child Maltreatment, 2020, Crimes Against Children Research Center, University of New Hampshire. 2022. Available at: https://www.unh.edu/ccrc/sites/default/files/media/2022-03/updated-trends-2020-final.pdf. Accessed July 26, 2023.

16. Hillis S, N'konzi JN, Msemburi W, et al. Orphanhood and Caregiver Loss Among Children Based on New Global Excess COVID-19 Death Estimates. JAMA Pediatr 2022;176(11):1145–8.

17. Andrade C, Gillen M, Molina JA, et al. The Social and Economic Impact of Covid-19 on Family Functioning and Well-Being: Where do we go from here? J Fam Econ Issues 2022;43(2):205–12.

18. He Y, Ortiz R, Kishton R, et al. In their own words: Child and adolescent perceptions of caregiver stress during early COVID-19. Child Abuse Negl 2022;124:105452.

19. Sinko L, He Y, Kishton R, et al. "The Stay at Home Order is Causing Things to Get Heated Up": Family Conflict Dynamics During COVID-19 From The Perspectives of Youth Calling a National Child Abuse Hotline. J Fam Violence 2022;37(5):837–46.

20. Ortiz R, Kishton R, Sinko L, et al. Assessing Child Abuse Hotline Inquiries in the Wake of COVID-19: Answering the Call. JAMA Pediatr 2021;175(8):859–61.

21. Rapp A, Fall G, Radomsky AC, et al. Child Maltreatment During the COVID-19 Pandemic: A Systematic Rapid Review. Pediatr Clin North Am 2021;68(5):991–1009.

22. Dettlaff AJ, Boyd R. Racial Disproportionality and Disparities in the Child Welfare System: Why Do They Exist, and What Can Be Done to Address Them? Ann Am Acad Polit Soc Sci 2020;692(1):253–74.

23. Minoff E and Citrin A. "Systemically Neglected: How Racism Structures Public Systems to Produce Child Neglect." Center for the Study of Social Policy, 2022. Available at: https://cssp.org/resource/systemically-neglected/. Accessed July 26, 2023.

24. Cénat JM, McIntee SE, Mukunzi JN, et al. Overrepresentation of Black children in the child welfare system: A systematic review to understand and better act. Child Youth Serv Rev 2021;120:105714.

25. Yi Y, Edwards FR, Wildeman C. Cumulative Prevalence of Confirmed Maltreatment and Foster Care Placement for US Children by Race/Ethnicity, 2011-2016. Am J Public Health 2020;110(5):704–9.

26. Child Welfare Information Gateway. (2021). Child welfare practice to address racial disproportionality and disparity. U.S. Department of Health and Human Services, Administration for Children and Families, Children's Bureau. Available at: https://www.childwelfare.gov/pubs/issue-briefs/racial-disproportionality/. Accessed July 26, 2023.

27. Lane WG, Rubin DM, Monteith R, et al. Racial differences in the evaluation of pediatric fractures for physical abuse. JAMA 2002;288(13):1603–9.

28. Hymel KP, Laskey AL, Crowell KR, et al. Racial and Ethnic Disparities and Bias in the Evaluation and Reporting of Abusive Head Trauma. J Pediatr 2018;198:137–43.e1.

29. He Y, Leventhal JM, Gaither JR, et al. Trends from 2005 to 2018 in child maltreatment outcomes with caregivers' substance use. Child Abuse Negl 2022;131:105781.

30. Jones CP. Levels of racism: a theoretic framework and a gardener's tale. Am J Public Health 2000;90(8):1212–5.

31. Children's Bureau. 2022. The AFCARS report: Preliminary FY 2021 estimates as of June 28, 2022 - No. 29. U.S. Department of Health and Human Services, Administration for Children and Families. Available at: https://www.acf.hhs.gov/sites/default/files/documents/cb/afcars-report-29.pdf. Accessed July 26, 2023.

32. Child Welfare Information Gateway. (2019). Mandatory reporters of child abuse and neglect. U.S. Department of Health and Human Services, Administration for

Children and Families, Children's Bureau. Available at: https://www.childwelfare. gov/topics/systemwide/laws-policies/statutes/manda/. Accessed July 26, 2023.

33. Sege RD, Flaherty EG. Forty years later: inconsistencies in reporting of child abuse. Arch Dis Child 2008;93(10):822–4.

34. Flaherty EG, Sege R, Binns HJ, et al. Health care providers' experience reporting child abuse in the primary care setting. Pediatric Practice Research Group. Arch Pediatr Adolesc Med 2000;154(5):489–93.

35. Flaherty EG, Sege R, Mattson CL, et al. Assessment of suspicion of abuse in the primary care setting. Ambul Pediatr 2002;2(2):120–6.

36. Flaherty EG, Jones R, Sege R, Child Abuse Recognition Experience Study Research Group. Telling their stories: primary care practitioners' experience evaluating and reporting injuries caused by child abuse. Child Abuse Negl 2004; 28(9):939–45.

37. Gunn VL, Hickson GB, Cooper WO. Factors affecting pediatricians' reporting of suspected child maltreatment. Ambul Pediatr 2005;5(2):96–101.

38. Flaherty EG, Sege RD, Griffith J, et al. From suspicion of physical child abuse to reporting: primary care clinician decision-making. Pediatrics 2008;122(3):611–9.

39. Lloyd MH, Akin BA, Brook J, et al. The Policy to Practice Gap: Factors Associated With Practitioner Knowledge of CAPTA 2010 Mandates for Identifying and Intervening in Cases of Prenatal Alcohol and Drug Exposure. Fam Soc 2023;99(3): 232–43.

40. Wood JN, Paine CW, La Rochelle C. Improving Child Physical Abuse Detection & Reducing Disparities Within and Between Hospital Settings. PolicyLab at Children's Hospital of Philadelphia; 2022. Available at: https://policylab.chop.edu/ sites/default/files/pdf/publications/PolicyLab-Evidence-to-Action-Brief-Improving-Child-Physical-Abuse-Detection.pdf. Accessed July 26, 2023.

41. Christian CW. Committee on Child Abuse and Neglect, American Academy of Pediatrics. The evaluation of suspected child physical abuse. Pediatrics 2015; 135(5):e1337–54.

42. Section on Radiology, American Academy of Pediatrics. Diagnostic imaging of child abuse. Pediatrics 2009;123(5):1430–5.

43. Narang SK, Fingarson A, Lukefahr J, et al. COUNCIL ON CHILD ABUSE AND NEGLECT. Abusive Head Trauma in Infants and Children. Pediatrics 2020; 145(4). https://doi.org/10.1542/peds.2020-0203.

44. Legano LA, Desch LW, Messner SA, et al. Maltreatment of Children With Disabilities. Pediatrics 2021;147(5). https://doi.org/10.1542/peds.2021-050920.

45. The City of Philadelphia Budget Office. Budgeting for Racial Equity, Fiscal Year 2023. Available at: https://www.phila.gov/media/20220330122553/FY2023-2027-Five-Year-Plan-Budgeting-for-Racial-Equity.pdf. Accessed July 26, 2023.

46. Forkey H, Szilagyi M, Kelly ET, et al. COUNCIL ON FOSTER CARE A, AND KINSHIP CARE, COUNCIL ON COMMUNITY PEDIATRICS, COUNCIL ON CHILD ABUSE AND NEGLECT, COMMITTEE ON PSYCHOSOCIAL ASPECTS OF CHILD AND FAMILY HEALTH. Trauma-Informed Care. Pediatrics 2021;148(2). https:// doi.org/10.1542/peds.2021-052580.

47. Flaherty E, Legano L, Idzerda S, et al, COUNCIL ON CHILD ABUSE AND NEGLECT. Ongoing Pediatric Health Care for the Child Who Has Been Maltreated. Pediatrics 2019;143(4). https://doi.org/10.1542/peds.2019-0284.

48. Fortson BL, Klevens J, Merrick MT, et al. Preventing child abuse and neglect: a technical package for policy, norm, and programmatic activities. Atlanta, GA: National Center for Injury Prevention and Control, Centers for Disease Control and Prevention; 2016.

49. Flaherty EG, Stirling J, American Academy of Pediatrics COUNCIL ON CHILD ABUSE AND NEGLECT. Clinical report—the pediatrician's role in child maltreatment prevention. Pediatrics 2010;126(4):833–41.
50. Center for the Study of Social Policy. Strengthening families: the protective factors framework. Accessed February 27, 2023, Available at: https://cssp.org/our-work/projects/protective-factors-framework/.
51. Greenthal E, Jia J, Poblacion A, et al. Patient experiences and provider perspectives on a hospital-based food pantry: a mixed methods evaluation study. Public Health Nutr 2019;22(17):3261–9.
52. Berry WS, Blatt SD. Diaper Need? You Can Bank on It. Acad Pediatr 2021;21(1): 188–9.
53. Beck AF, Henize AW, Qiu T, et al. Reductions In Hospitalizations Among Children Referred To A Primary Care-Based Medical-Legal Partnership. Health Aff 2022; 41(3):341–9.
54. Marcil LE, Hole MK, Jackson J, et al. Anti-Poverty Medicine Through Medical-Financial Partnerships: A New Approach to Child Poverty. Acad Pediatr 2021; 21(8S):S169–76.
55. Saoud K, Saavedra J, Hirshfield LE, et al. Addressing Barriers to Accessing Head Start Programs via the Medical Home: A Qualitative Study. Matern Child Health J 2022;26(10):2118–25.
56. Atkins DN, Durrance CP. State Policies That Treat Prenatal Substance Use As Child Abuse Or Neglect Fail To Achieve Their Intended Goals. Health Aff 2020; 39(5):756–63.
57. Bullinger LR, Fong K. Evictions and Neighborhood Child Maltreatment Reports. Housing Policy Debate 2021;31(3–5):490–515.
58. Coulton CJ, Crampton DS, Irwin M, et al. How neighborhoods influence child maltreatment: a review of the literature and alternative pathways. Child Abuse Negl 2007;31(11–12):1117–42.
59. Klevens J, Schmidt B, Luo F, et al. Effect of the Earned Income Tax Credit on Hospital Admissions for Pediatric Abusive Head Trauma, 1995-2013. Public Health Rep 2017;132(4):505–11.
60. Kovski NL, Hill HD, Mooney SJ, et al. Association of State-Level Earned Income Tax Credits With Rates of Reported Child Maltreatment, 2004-2017. Child Maltreat 2022;27(3):325–33.
61. Kovski NL, Hill HD, Mooney SJ, et al. Short-Term Effects of Tax Credits on Rates of Child Maltreatment Reports in the United States. Pediatrics 2022;150(1). https://doi.org/10.1542/peds.2021-054939.

Bullying and School Violence

Daniel J. Flannery, PhD[a],*, Seth J. Scholer, MD[b],
Ivette Noriega, PhD[a]

KEYWORDS

- Bullying • Cyber bullying • Bullying victimization • School violence
- Vulnerable youth • Mental health

KEY POINTS

- Rates of traditional bullying have remained stable (30%) but rates of cyberbullying are increasing rapidly (46% of youth).
- There are significant long-term physical and mental health consequences of bullying especially for vulnerable youth.
- Multi-component school-based prevention programs that include caring adults, positive school climate, and supportive services for involved youth can effectively reduce bullying.
- While bullying has emerged as a legitimate concern, studies of surviving perpetrators to date suggest bullying is not the most significant risk factor of mass school shootings.
- Pediatricians play a critical role in identification, intervention, awareness, and advocacy.

INTRODUCTION AND BACKGROUND

While historically perceived to be part of the normal rite of passage growing up, bullying is now recognized as a significant but preventable public health problem, and pediatricians play an important role in its identification, prevention, and intervention. The consequences of bullying, for those who are bullied, those who witness bullying, and for those who perpetrate bullying, include poor physical health, and poor mental health such as increased anxiety, depression and increased risk for suicide. Youth who experience bullying are also at increased risk of poor school performance and future delinquent and aggressive behavior.[1–3] A significant challenge is the

To appear in: Fein, J., & Bair-Merritt, M. (Eds). Addressing violence in pediatric practice. *Pediatric Clinics of North America*.

[a] Begun Center for Violence Prevention, Research and Education, Jack, Joseph and Morton Mandel School of Applied Social Sciences, Case Western Reserve University, 11402 Bellflower Boulevard, Cleveland, OH 44102, USA; [b] Vanderbilt University Medical Center, D0T8 2200 Childrens Way, Nashville, TN 37232, USA
* Corresponding author. Mandel School of Applied Social Sciences, Case Western Reserve University, 11402 Bellflower Boulevard, Cleveland, OH 44102.
E-mail address: djf6@case.edu

Pediatr Clin N Am 70 (2023) 1153–1170
https://doi.org/10.1016/j.pcl.2023.06.014
0031-3955/23/© 2023 Elsevier Inc. All rights reserved.

increase in cyberbullying driven by more frequent use and exposure to social media in its varied forms and platforms. A comprehensive panel study report on bullying by the National Academies of Sciences, Engineering, and Medicine[4] laid out what was known about bullying at the time, but since then we have learned even more about the various manifestations of bullying, which types of preventive interventions are most effective to address bullying victimization and perpetration, and important protective factors.[5–7] We review below issues of particular importance to pediatricians, including the changing nature of bullying, the increased importance of cyberbullying, understanding how to identify risk and protective factors for bullying, and how to prevent or intervene to address bullying for children and adolescents.

Definition

The definition of bullying behavior varies depending on who is addressing the issue. Researchers define bullying differently than lawmakers, and reported incidence and prevalence rates of bullying will vary depending on the definition and method used to gather the information. The formal definition of bullying adopted by the Centers for Disease Control and Prevention is.

- Bullying is any unwanted aggressive behavior(s) by another youth or group of youths who are not siblings or current dating partners that involves an observed or perceived power imbalance and is repeated multiple times or is highly likely to be repeated.

Bullying may inflict harm or distress on the targeted youth including physical, psychological, social, or educational harm.[4]

However, almost nobody uses the formal definition adopted by the CDC when they ask youth about their experiences with bullying. A typical question is "have you ever been bullied?" or some other general reference, leaving it up to the reporter to determine what bullying means for him or her. Clearly definitions matter, particularly how they impact our understanding of changing incidence and prevalence rates of different and emerging types of bullying. For example, peer victimization is a term often used interchangeably with bullying in the literature, but a single incident of victimization would not meet the formal criteria of traditional bullying where repeated behaviors are required.

The changing landscape of bullying complicates how the behavior is identified, assessed, and addressed. Bullying in school has been traditionally defined in relational and physical terms.[8] More recently we have recognized that bullying does not always occur directly between two persons with a physical altercation, but can be indirect or relational (spreading rumors, rejection), and can occur via social media or in on-line forums, where no obvious power imbalance may be evident. The latter is most referred to as cyberbullying, which is different than traditional forms of bullying. A single post on social media (vs repeated incidents) can be anonymous (vs an identified power imbalance) and go viral quickly resulting in significant harm to the intended target.[9]

Developmentally, bullying behavior is evident as early as preschool, although it typically peaks during the middle school years.[10,11] It can occur in diverse social settings, including classrooms, school gyms and cafeterias, on school buses, and online. Bullying behavior affects not only the children and youth who are bullied or bully others, but also bystanders to bullying incidents. Given the myriad situations in which bullying can occur and the many people who may be involved, identifying effective prevention programs and policies is critical, yet challenging; it is unlikely that any one approach will be appropriate in all situations or effective for all youth. This is especially true as we move beyond a focus on the victims of bullying to better understand those who perpetrate bullying and bully-victims.[12]

The Scope of the Problem

Research suggests disparities in rates of bullying by a variety of individual characteristics, including sexual orientation, disability, and obesity, though there is a lack of nationally representative data on these and other vulnerable groups. Estimated prevalence rates for bullying and cyberbullying vary greatly, ranging from 17.9% to 30.9% of school-aged children for frequency of bullying behavior at school and from 6.9% to 14.8% for the prevalence of cyberbullying,[13–15] though recently as much as 46% of youth report being victims of cyberbullying,[16] and approximately one-third of youth who are cyberbullied also report being victims of traditional bullying.[17–19]

The prevalence of bullying victimization is even higher for anybody who stands out as being different, which increases the risk of bullying victimization. For instance, the prevalence of bullying of lesbian, gay, bisexual, and transgender (LGBTQ) youth is approximately double that of heterosexual and cisgender youth.[4,20,21] Youth with chronic health conditions are also more likely to be victims of bullying than their peers including children who are overweight, children with autism spectrum disorder, and youth diagnosed with ADHD. Even children with food allergies and epilepsy have reported higher rates of bullying victimization.[22] One challenge is that most previous studies of bullying have focused primarily on children who are bullied. Considerably less is known about perpetrators, and very little is known about bullying's impact on bystanders in the national data.

Social Context

At the individual level, we know that boys are at greater risk of being physically bullied and girls are at greater risk of being emotionally or cyberbullied,[23] but social context matters because bullying affects and is affected by peers, families, schools, and communities.[1,24] Each of these contexts interact with individual characteristics of youth (eg, race/ethnicity, sexual orientation) in ways that either exacerbate or attenuate the association between these individual characteristics and perpetrating and/or being the target of bullying behavior. Cyberbullying is particularly difficult for schools to control or address, especially if the behavior does not occur on school grounds or with school equipment.[25]

Traditional bullying is conceptualized as a group phenomenon, with multiple peers taking on roles other than perpetrator and target. Cyberbullying can also be perpetrated by multiple persons or observed by multiple peers. Thus peers are a critical social context that affects many aspects of bullying—in large part because peers influence group norms, attitudes, and behavior. The peer group context is important to consider, given what is known about factors associated with bullying, whether one is concerned about in person or cyberbullying. For example, having friends and being liked by peers can protect children against being bullied, and having a high-quality best friendship might help protect children from being targets of bullying behavior. Families also play an important role in bullying prevention, as family functioning and support have been linked to whether a child is identified as one who engages in bullying perpetration or one who is the target of bullying behavior.[26] A recent meta-analysis showed that self-oriented personal competence was the strongest protective factor against victimization, while low technology use was the most protective of involvement in cyberbullying.[27] Good academic performance and other-oriented social competencies guarded best against being a bully-victim.

Bullying behavior has most often been studied in the school context. The organization of instruction, discipline practices, classroom norms, the ethnic composition of classrooms and schools, and teacher behavior are several factors at the school level that have been shown to moderate the effect of individual characteristics on bullying outcomes. A school's instructional practices such as grouping students together can worsen the experience of bullying by limiting student exposure to the larger school community. For example, Echols,[28] found that, for students who were not well liked by their peers, grouping students together into small teams *increased* the experience of being bullied by their peers. In other words, socially vulnerable adolescents who were traveling with the same classmates throughout most of the school day were found to have few opportunities to redefine their social identities or change their status among peers. Regarding the ethnic composition of schools, youth who are members of ethnic or religious minority groups are at greater risk for being bullied especially if they have fewer same ethnicity peers to help ward off potential perpetrators.[29] Last, schools' discipline climate is associated with individuals' risk of being bullied as well as the amount of bullying that occurs.[4] In both the United States and internationally the evidence consistently shows that rates of bullying behavior are highest in schools with poor discipline and where teachers treat students unfairly, while schools with a positive and supportive school climate report lower rates of bullying perpetration and victimization.[4,30]

Consequences of Bullying Behavior

Bullying has significant short- and long-term internalizing and externalizing psychological consequences for the children who are involved in bullying behavior (**Table 1**).[31] Mounting evidence has highlighted the detrimental effects of being bullied on children's health and behavior.[32–35] The physical health consequences of bullying can be immediate, such as physical injury, or they can involve long-term effects, such as headaches, sleep disturbances, or somatization.[36] However, long-term physical consequences can be difficult to identify and link with past bullying behavior, as they can also be the result of other causes such as anxiety or other adverse childhood events.[37,38]

Psychological problems are also common after being bullied.[39] and include internalizing problems such as depression, anxiety, and especially for girls, self-harming behavior.[31,40,41] Youth who are bullied often have low self-esteem and feel depressed, anxious, and lonely.[42] There can also be subsequent externalizing behavior problems, especially for boys.[31] Recent longitudinal studies have shown the effects of childhood

Table 1 Adverse outcomes associated with bullying		
Bullying Victim	**Bully-Victim**	**Bullying Perpetrator**
Depression	Anxiety disorders	Aggressive behavior
Somatic complaints	Depression	Delinquent behavior
Anxiety disorders	Poor health	Conduct disorder
Social relationship problems	Lower academic performance	Antisocial personality disorder
Poor physical health	Social relationship problems	Criminal offending
Decreased lifetime wealth	Decreased lifetime wealth	
Lower academic performance	Suicidal ideation and attempts	
Sleep problems		
Suicidal ideation and attempts		

bullying on adult mental health were stronger in magnitude than the effects of being maltreated by a caregiver in childhood.[33]

Some meta-analyses have examined the association between involvement in bullying and internalizing problems in the school-aged population and concluded that individuals who are both perpetrators and targets of bullying (eg, bully-victims) had a significantly higher risk for psychosomatic problems than individuals who were only perpetrators or who were only targets.[32,34] In their meta-analysis, Gini and Pozzoli[32] reviewed studies that examined the association between involvement in bullying and psychosomatic complaints in children and adolescents. They found that individuals who bully and are also bullied by others have a significantly higher risk for psychosomatic problems than uninvolved peers. Other meta-analyses found in longitudinal studies that internalizing emotional problems increase both the risk and the harmful consequences of being bullied.[34,43] Individuals who bully and who are also bullied by others are especially at risk for suicidal ideation and behavior, due to increased mental health problems.[44] Individuals who bully others and are themselves bullied also appear to be at greatest risk for poor psychosocial outcomes, compared to those who only bully or are only bullied, and to those who are not bullied.[45]

Individuals who have been cyberbullied report higher levels of depression and suicidal ideation, as well as increased emotional distress, externalized hostility, and delinquency, compared with peers who were not bullied.[46] Severity of depression in youth who have been cyberbullied has also been shown to correlate with the degree and severity of cyberbullying.[37]

Several studies have documented links between being bullied and violence or crime, especially for men.[47–50] A meta-analysis that included studies with data on 5825 participants showed that after controlling for externalizing symptoms at baseline, peer victimization—under which they included being the target of teasing, deliberate exclusion, and being the target of physical threats and malicious gossip—was associated over time with exhibiting externalizing problems such as aggression, truancy, and delinquency.[49] Reijntjes and colleagues[51] found that externalizing problems predicted changes in peer victimization over time and concluded that there is a bidirectional relationship between peer victimization and externalizing problems.

Although the effects of bullying on brain development and function are not yet fully understood, there are known to be changes in the stress response systems that are associated with increased risk of mental health problems, cognitive function, self-regulation, and other physical health problems (NAS, 2016).[4] One topic that has received recent attention is the possible association of bullying victimization and risk for the perpetration of school or mass shootings. While bullying has emerged as a legitimate concern, studies of surviving perpetrators or intensive psychological autopsy assessments post-incident suggest bullying is not the most significant risk factor nor is it presently viewed as predictive of mass shootings.[19,52,53] Pediatricians should be aware that many schools have implemented threat assessment teams as a strategy to address the continuum of aggressive or violent behaviors that can impact a school, and how community providers might contribute to assessments of students deemed to be of concern due to their involvement in bullying.[54–56]

Preventive Interventions

The research on bullying prevention programming has increased considerably over the past two decades, which is likely due in part to the growing awareness of bullying as a public health problem. Despite this growing interest, there have been relatively few randomized controlled trials (RCTs) testing the efficacy or effectiveness of programs specifically designed to reduce or prevent the onset of bullying or offset its consequences for children and youth.[57,58] Moreover, the much larger body and longer line of research focused on aggression, violence, delinquent behavior or externalizing problems has only recently begun to explore program impacts specific to bullying.[57]

The most effective bullying prevention programs are whole school, multicomponent programs that combine elements of universal and targeted strategies.[4,57] Programs are more effective when they are implemented with fidelity to program guidelines rather than being adapted in non-systematic ways to specific school conditions.[59] Programs in schools also work better if they address the social environment and the broader culture and climate of bullying.[60] For example, research documents the importance of school-wide prevention efforts that provide positive behavior support, establish a common set of expectations for positive behavior across all school contexts, and involve all school staff in prevention activities.[61] Effective supervision, especially in bullying "hot spots," such as the playground, and clear anti-bullying policies are essential elements of a successful school-wide prevention effort.[62–64] Data from anonymous student surveys can identify potential areas for intensive training of school staff, also an essential element of successful efforts.[62]

A meta-analyses of the effectiveness of school-based bullying prevention programs found that bullying perpetration rates can be reduced by about 20% and victimization by about 15%, with the most favorable results for studies that focus on age-appropriate preventive interventions with more rigorous research designs.[6] Gaffney and colleagues[65] found that anti-cyberbullying programs can reduce cyberbullying perpetration by about 9% to 15% and cyberbullying victimization by about 14% to 15%. There is also emerging evidence that programs are more effective for younger children in elementary or middle school compared to youth in high school.[66,67]

Families also play a critical role in bullying prevention by providing emotional support to promote disclosure of bullying incidents and by fostering coping skills in their children. Parents may need training in how to talk with their children about bullying,[68] how to communicate their concerns about bullying to the school, and how to get actively involved in school-based bullying prevention efforts.[69] There also are important bullying prevention activities that can occur at the community level, such as awareness or social marketing campaigns that encourage all youth and adults to intervene when they see bullying and to become actively involved in school- and community-based prevention activities.[4,9]

A public health approach to bullying prevention works best but few bullying programs include specific intervention components for youth at risk for involvement in bullying or for youth already involved in bullying, whether as perpetrators or targets (or both). Few of the selective and indicated preventive interventions for identified perpetrators (aggressive youth) or targets (youth with mental health issues or at risk for suicide) are school-based, so there needs to be stronger connections between schools, families, and community-based treatment programs. The focus of these interventions tends to be on other behavioral concerns such as aggression or mental health problems, not bullying specifically, that co-occur and have overlapping risk and protective factors, which suggests these other evidence-based selective and indicated violence prevention models may also demonstrate positive effects for youth involved in bullying.[57]

There remains a dearth of intervention research on programs related to cyberbullying and on programs targeted to vulnerable populations such as LGBTQ youth, youth with chronic health problems, or youth with developmental disabilities such as autism.[70] The role of peers in interventions for at-risk students or for those who are perpetrators or targets needs further clarification, whether that is for peers as bystanders or peers as interventionists, or peers as fellow perpetrators, or targets. There has also been recent work utilizing technology to deliver bullying prevention materials and programs via social media, video games, and virtual reality that deserve increased attention relative to programs that address more traditional forms of bullying.[71]

Addressing Bullying in Pediatric Practice

Pediatric health care providers are uniquely positioned to play a significant role in addressing bullying. They see children and adolescents for annual well visits and acute care visits during the peak ages for bullying. Pediatricians are trained to focus on multiple health domains (eg, medical, psychosocial), understand the associations between exposures (ie, involvement in bullying) and adverse health outcomes (ie, internalizing problems), and trauma-informed care. Related to bullying, pediatricians are experts in advocating for their patients (eg, empowering families to involve the school system) and, as indicated, elevating the level of care (eg, referring a youth with anxieties for a mental health assessment).

While researchers have made headway with understanding the effects of bullying interventions in schools, research of office-based approaches to address bullying is lacking, likely because of the many confounders that researchers would need to consider to conduct such studies. There are many variations for how a youth involved in bullying might present, often with factors that are difficult to measure. Some youth involved in bullying may present with somatic complaints and, even after extensive questioning, may deny being bullied. Other youth may present to the office with the chief complaint of being bullied yet, upon further questioning and considering the definition of bullying, it is determined that the youth is experiencing what most people would consider normal peer to peer interactions (eg, teasing). Health care providers will need a different approach for youth who have been bullied compared to youth who engage in bullying behavior. In an office-based study, it would be important to control for the home and school environment. It is unclear whether researchers will be able to overcome the barriers and confounders to conduct studies in pediatric

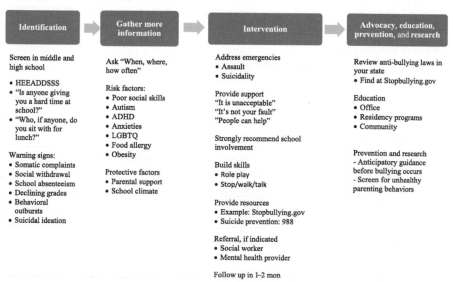

Fig. 1. A systematic approach to address bullying in pediatric primary care.

primary care. For now, we present a systematic approach that includes important public health activities: identification, information gathering, intervention, advocacy, education, and prevention (**Fig. 1**).

IDENTIFICATION

As with any disease or condition, a thoughtful first step is identification which, for bullying, should include attention to warning signs and routine screening (**Table 2**). For the child who is being bullied, common somatic complaints are abdominal pain, headaches, fatigue, heart palpitations, dizziness, and incontinence.[72] These complaints are also potentially associated with mood disorders. A child who is being bullied may also present with school absenteeism, declining grades, or suicidal ideation. Children who have been cyberbullied might have a change in behavior or mood, especially after spending time on a device. It is easier for health care providers to identify warning signs for victims of bullying than for those who are perpetrators of bullying. A parent of a child who bullies may report that their child uses physical or verbal aggression to resolve conflicts, blames others, or arrives home with items that do not belong to them.

Screening questions can also help identify children involved in bullying. One bullying-specific screen has 8 questions for youth and 5 for parents.[73] Another screening tool has been developed for use in the emergency department.[74] Screening for bullying can also be done through routine intake forms such as the AAP Bright Futures Questionnaire.[75] A screening tool familiar to many providers that can illicit bullying involvement is the HEEADSSS assessment–the E stands for education, S for suicidal ideation, and S for Safety. Pertinent education questions related are, "How do you get along with others at school?" or "How many days of school did you miss last year?" A suicidal ideation question might be, "Have you had thoughts about hurting yourself or wishing you were not alive?" An example of a safety question is, "Do other students pick on you at school?" When screening for bullying, providers should consider that approximately 70% of youth who are bullied do not want to admit that they are being bullied. Therefore, it may be best to avoid the loaded term, "bullying," and consider using a roundabout approach to screen for bullying. Examples include:

"How is school going?"
"Who, if anyone, do you sit with for lunch?"
"Is anyone giving you a hard time at school?"

Table 2 Warning signs	
Youth Who Are Bullied	**Youth Who Bullies**
Somatic complaints	Uses verbal or physical aggression to address conflict
Anxieties	Blames others for behavior
Depression	Comes home with items that do not belong to them.
Social withdrawal	
School absenteeism	
Declining grades	
Behavioral outbursts	
Suicidal ideation	

"Do you ever feel afraid to go to school?"

GATHER MORE INFORMATION

If there is a suspicion for bullying, the second step is to gather more information (see **Fig. 1**). Many people do not understand the definition of bullying. Therefore, do not assume that if a child says they were bullied, they were. Listen to the child–asking what happened, when, and where. Has the event happened once or multiple times? Is there a power imbalance? Did the event(s) occur on the school bus, in the locker room, or on social media? From this information, the provider can determine whether the behaviors represent bullying or some other type of conflict. Some children are affected more profoundly by bullying than others so providers should consider asking how the events have affected the child (eg, behavior, somatic symptoms, grades, school attendance, relationships).

As the provider gathers more information, this is an opportune time to reflect on risk and protective factors (see **Fig. 1**) and maybe even inquire about school climate, especially whether the school has antibullying policies that include sexual orientation. Of note, there is no single risk or protective factor that results in involvement in bullying. This is because of the complex interactions of individual, family, and community factors. For example, a boy with poor social skills who has supportive parents and who attends a school with policies that prohibit bullying may be less likely to be bullied than a boy with poor social skills who has parents with unhealthy parenting behaviors and who attends a school that does not have antibullying education and policies. A girl exposed to unhealthy parenting (eg, physical punishment, humiliation) or domestic violence may be more likely to bully.

INTERVENTION
What Doesn't Work

Before intervening, health care providers should be aware of interventions that either *do not work* or that could make the situation worse (**Table 3**).

Is it an Emergency?

Most cases of bullying are not emergencies; still, an important early decision is whether the situation might rise to that level (see **Fig. 1**). If there is imminent danger or there was an assault, either physical or sexual, then duty to warn may require that you contact law enforcement. If there are concerns about suicidality or homicidality, contact a mental health professional or, as indicated, transport the youth to the nearest emergency department. When no emergency exists, the provider can proceed systematically as outlined later in discussion or, if there are time constraints, provide a brief intervention and reschedule for a dedicated appointment (see section on "Addressing bullying and office time constraints").

Support

Health care providers should start by offering support. For example, ensure that youth understand that it is not their fault and that there are, almost always, people who want to help at home and at school.

School Involvement

Schools are where most bullying events occur and should be involved in the solution. If not done already, youth and their families should be encouraged to communicate the concern with the school. Realizing that addressing bullying can take time, parents

Table 3	
Responses that, in general, do not work to address bullying	
Responses to Avoid	**Comments**
Ignoring	Ignoring the situation or thinking of bullying as "rite of passage" may result in prolonged exposure to a risk factor, bullying, that is known to be associated with adverse outcomes.
Blaming the child	Blaming the child who was bullied may perpetuate feelings of shame and decrease the likelihood that the child will reach out to adults for help in the future. Blaming the child who bullies is also an ineffective remedy.
Peer mediation	Peer mediation may be appropriate for other interpersonal disputes but should not be used for bullying because of the perceived power imbalance.
Retaliation	Retaliation should not be used as it is likely to escalate hurtful behaviors.
School suspension	School suspension and "zero tolerance policies" have, in general, been found to be counterproductive as they may lead to indiscriminate, sometimes arbitrary, suspensions or expulsions. Also, these policies can hinder academic progress for at-risk youth, especially when students are suspended without other school or community supports.
Calling the parents	Parents of the child who was bullied should not contact the parents of the child who has engaged in the bullying behavior; rather, the school should investigate and make contact as indicated.
Taking away a device	Taking away a smart phone is not advised because youth will be less likely to report cyberbullying in the future if they know that their device may be taken.

should be empowered to continue working with the school until the issue is resolved. If teachers and school counselors are not responsive after a reasonable amount of time, parents can consider contacting higher level administrators such as the principal or superintendent.

Build Skills–Traditional Bullying

All youth should develop skills to respond to others when they are hurt–youth who have been bullied will likely need extra support in this area. A recognized way to build skills is through role play. Let youth know that everyone needs practice dealing with challenging situations that require quick, effective responses. Essentially, a caring adult asks the child who was bullied what they are going to do the next time it occurs. Health care providers can do role play in the office and, because repetition helps, parents can be encouraged to practice role play at home.

Recognizing that every bullying situation is different, youth who are bullied can learn basic principles of responding to bullying by memorizing three words, "Stop," "Walk," and "Talk."

- "Stop": Youth should speak to bullies with direct eye contact, brevity, and confidence, telling the child who bullied to "stop" in a firm voice. "Stop" can be replaced with other words such as, "enough," "that's overboard," "too far," "not cool."
- "Walk": Youth should walk away, not run, from the situation with confidence (ie, with head held high and good posture). They should not linger for more abuse to potentially occur. Retaliation typically escalates the situation.

- "Talk": Children should be encouraged to talk to a parent, school counselor, or teacher. Explain to the child, "Telling an adult can help you feel less alone, and adults can help you make a plan to stop the bullying."

Another skill building exercise is to encourage the child to actively seek out other friendships. This can be particularly helpful for children with poor social skills.

Build Skills–Cyberbullying

Cyberbullying requires a different set of skills in the areas of both prevention and response. An important modality to prevent cyberbullying is digital citizenship. Encourage parents to have discussions about online behaviors and real-world consequences. During everyday conversations, parents can ask questions such as.

- "What do you know about cyberbullying?"
- "What are you doing to keep yourself safe?"
- "Do you pause before you post?"

To respond to cyberbullying, youth should consider.

- Don't respond, forward, or "Like" posts.
- Keep the evidence: Dates, times, descriptions, screen shots, emails, and texts.
- Consider blocking the person who is cyberbullying.
- Talk to a trusted adult. If indicated, parents should help with reporting to the online service provider or content provider, law enforcement (eg, threats of violence, child pornography, stalking, hate crimes), or the school.

Intervention for the Child Who Bullies

Although health care providers will, most often, identify children who have been bullied, they might also identify a child who has bullying behavior. In this situation, the intervention will need to mostly be at the level of the parent. This is often a delicate matter because some parents of youth who have been bullying may not want to accept that it is a problem. The health care provider might take a moment to explain the adverse consequences of involvement in bullying (see **Table 2**). Once everyone is in agreement that an intervention is needed, recommendations can include the following: setting firm limits (eg, "bullying is never OK"); encourage the use of healthy discipline; working with teachers and school counselors; and, if indicated, refer for counseling with a focus on anger management and effective coping and problem solving skills.

Provide Resources

Providing resources is an important step in helping the child and their family gain a better understanding of bullying. There are many resources available. One of the best is www.stopbullying.gov/, a comprehensive online resource with information about traditional bullying, cyberbullying, risk groups, how to prevent bullying, how to respond to bullying, state anti-bullying laws and policies, and links to resources. Some youth exposed to bullying have self-injurious thoughts; as indicated, health care providers can let youth know about the National Suicide Prevention Lifeline, 988.

Referral

Referral will depend upon the circumstances and your local resources. If internalizing risk factors are identified (eg, anxieties, depression) during screening, the health care provider might refer to a mental health professional for confirmation and therapy as indicated (eg, cognitive behavior therapy). For poor social skills, it may be helpful for the child to receive counseling in the area of social skills training and problem solving. For autism, applied behavioral analysis may be helpful.

Follow up

The health care provider can recommend a follow up visit in 1 to 2 months, sending a strong message that bullying is unacceptable and needs to be resolved.

ADVOCACY, EDUCATION, AND PREVENTION

Pediatric health care providers who are interested in additional steps to address bullying may want to consider advocacy, education, and prevention strategies (see **Fig. 1**).

Advocacy

All states have either laws or policies designed to prevent bullying in schools, but the strength of the laws vary from state to state. Pediatricians can consider partnering with schools and policy makers to strengthen antibullying laws and working with community leaders to improve services to counsel youth who are involved in bullying. Primary care providers are encouraged to learn more about what can be done through documents published by the US Department of Health and Human Services, the US Department of Education, the National Academy of Medicine, and other resources. Stopbullying.gov has an interactive map in which one can click on a state and be directed to that state's laws and policies related to bullying.[76]

Education

Education is a key component to decreasing many health problems, including bullying. Health care providers can contribute through educational efforts in the office, the community, and medical school and residency curricula.

Prevention

Efforts are needed to determine if office-based interventions can affect rates of bullying. One untapped example is for providers to think of bullying as other health problems for which they give anticipatory guidance. Similar to recommending a bicycle helmet for children who are approaching the age at which they might start riding a bike, anticipatory guidance recommendations related to bullying prevention could include routinely delivered messages to the parents of young children. For example, *"Mom, I want to take a minute to talk about bullying. Unfortunately, many children are bullied, either in person or electronically, also called cyberbullying. There is good news in that there are ways to decrease bullying. To help teach your child more about bullying and what to do if bullied or if they witness bullying as a bystander, please check out the website, Stopbullying.gov. Also, most children, almost three-quarters, never tell an adult. Let your child know that you are there to support them and help make a plan if they are ever involved in bullying."* Essentially, anticipatory guidance messages, delivered in the office to prepare youth to respond appropriately when they are involved in bullying, may help to extinguish bullying behaviors in their nascency.

Another idea is to reduce the number of children who develop bullying behaviors by building parenting skills in pediatric primary care. There is strong evidence that unhealthy parenting behaviors, such as overly coercive and derisive parenting, and unhealthy relationships at home can lead to bullying.[13,77] Health care providers could assess and intervene for unhealthy parenting before it contributes to a child's bullying behavior. Validated parenting assessment tools have been developed and integrated

---

Box 1
When there are time constraints, sample scripts for a 1-2 minute, office- based, intervention to help youth who are bullied

Offer support: "I am sorry to hear that you are being bullied. Bullying is a common problem that involves 20-30% of students. That doesn't make it right. In fact, it is unacceptable because it can affect people's health. Being bullied is not your fault! People in your life can help you, at home and at school."

School involvement: "Schools have policies to address bullying and want to be involved. If you have not already done it, please start by letting your teachers and school counselor know about the situation. Realize that it may take the school some time to gather information and respond."

Provide resources: "Everyone involved should learn ways to address bullying. One of the best resources is www.Stopbullying.gov. This website has information for everyone involved. Please check it out."

Follow up: "I would like to see you back in the office in a month or two to see how things are going and make sure we are not missing anything."

---

into practice.[78] Studies are needed to determine whether parenting assessment instruments could help providers address unhealthy parenting strategies before they contribute to a child's bullying behavior.

Addressing bullying and office time constraints
It is common for new health problems to be identified during a well visit. If pressed for time, health care providers can, in a minute or two, consider scripts to begin the process of resolving the bullying situation (**Box 1**). This approach gives the school time to address the issue and allows health care providers the opportunity to have a dedicated visit to build skills, screen more thoroughly for risk factors and refer as indicated.

In summary, a systematic approach to address bullying in primary care includes screening, gathering information, and intervening (see **Fig. 1**). Depending upon a providers' level of interest in addressing bullying, they can also be involved in advocacy, education, and prevention efforts. Providers will often identify bullying during a well visit when time is limited; in this situation, consider a 1 to 2 minute intervention and follow up in clinic for a dedicated visit to address the youth's individual situation more thoroughly (see **Box 1**). If this type of approach can be scaled up, pediatric primary care providers may be able to play a larger role in reducing the rates of adverse health problems associated with bullying.

CLINICS CARE POINTS

- Bullying is associated with many adverse outcomes; thus, it should not be ignored or thought of as a "rite of passage" to be endured.

- Most children who are bullied do not tell an adult.

- Addressing bullying in the office should be individualized–a systematic approach includes identification (eg, HEEADDSSS assessment), gathering more information (eg, screen for risk factors), and intervention (eg, skill building).

- Prevention efforts should be explored, including introducing routine anticipatory guidance messages and screening for unhealthy parenting.

- When there are time constraints, health care providers can take a minute or two to offer support, encourage school involvement, provide resources (eg, www.stopbullying.gov), and recommend follow-up in clinic at a later date for a more thorough assessment.

FINANCIAL DISCLOSURE

The authors have no financial conflicts of interest to report.

REFERENCES

1. Brewer SL Jr, Brewer HJ, Kulik KS. Bullying Victimization in Schools: Why the Whole School, Whole Community, Whole Child Model Is Essential. J Sch Health 2018;88(11):794–802. https://doi.org/10.1111/josh.12686.
2. Samara M, Da Silva Nascimento B, El-Asam A, et al. How Can Bullying Victimisation Lead to Lower Academic Achievement? A Systematic Review and Meta-Analysis of the Mediating Role of Cognitive-Motivational Factors. Int J Environ Res Publ Health 2021;18(5):2209.
3. Walters GD, Espelage DL. Bullying perpetration and subsequent delinquency: A regression–based analysis of early adolescent schoolchildren. J Early Adolesc 2019;39(5):669–88.
4. Flannery DJ, Todres J, Bradshaw CP, et al. Bullying Prevention: A Summary of the Report of the National Academies of Sciences, Engineering, and Medicine: Committee on the Biological and Psychosocial Effects of Peer Victimization: Lessons for Bullying Prevention. Prev Sci 2016;17(8):1044–53.
5. Cross D, Runions KC, Shaw T, et al. Friendly Schools Universal Bullying Prevention Intervention: Effectiveness with Secondary School Students. Int Journal of Bullying Prevention 2019;1:45–57.
6. Gaffney H, Farrington DP, Ttofi MM. Examining the Effectiveness of School-Bullying Intervention Programs Globally: a Meta-analysis. Int Journal of Bullying Prevention 2019;1:14–31.
7. Mandira MR, Stoltz T. Bullying risk and protective factors among elementary school students over time: A systematic review. Int J Educ Res 2021;109:101838.
8. What is Bullying? Stopbullying.gov. Updated June 30, 2022. Available at: https://www.stopbullying.gov/bullying/what-is-bullying. Accessed on February 24, 2023.
9. Bass PF, Scholer SJ, Flannery DJ, et al. How to identify and treat bullying. Contemp Pediatr 2019;36(6):30–4.
10. Currie C, Zanotti C, Morgan A, et al. Social determinants of health and well-being among young people. Copenhagen, Denmark: World Health Organization Regional Office for Europe; 2012.
11. Vaillancourt T, Trinh V, McDougall P, et al. Optimizing population screening of bullying in school-aged children. J Sch Violence 2010;9(3):233–50.
12. Smith PK. Bullying: Definition, Types, Causes, Consequences and Intervention. Social and Personality Psychology Compass 2016;10:519–32.
13. Fast Fact: Preventing Bullying. Centers for Disease Control and Prevention. Updated September 2, 2021. Available at: https://www.cdc.gov/violenceprevention/youthviolence/bullyingresearch/fastfact.html. Accessed January 6, 2023.
14. Bullying Statistics. Stopbullying.gov. Updated September 9, 2021. Available at: https://www.stopbullying.gov/resources/facts#_Fast_Facts. Accessed February 24, 2023.
15. National Center for Education Statistics. Bullying at school and electronic bullying. Condition of education. U.S. Department of Education, Institute of

Education Sciences; 2021. Available at: https://nces.ed.gov/programs/coe/indicator/a10. Accessed February 24, 2023.

16. Vogels EA. Teens and cyberbullying 2022. Pew Research Center; 2022. Available at: https://www.pewresearch.org/internet/2022/12/15/teens-and-cyberbullying-2022/. Accessed on February 20, 2023.

17. Schneider SK, O'Donnell L, Stueve A, et al. Cyberbullying, school bullying, and psychological distress: a regional census of high school students. Am J Public Health 2012;102(1):171–7.

18. Timmons-Mitchell J, Flannery DJ. What Pediatricians Should Know and Do about Cyberbullying. Pediatr Rev 2020;41(7):373–5.

19. Timmons-Mitchell J, Noriega I, Flannery DJ. Bullying in school and cyberspace. Oxford Research Encyclopedia of Criminology; 2021.

20. Berlan ED, Corliss HL, Field AE, et al. Sexual orientation and bullying among adolescents in the growing up today study. J Adolesc Health 2010;46(4):366–71. https://doi.org/10.1016/j.jadohealth.2009.10.015.

21. Olsen EO, Kann L, Vivolo-Kantor A, et al. School violence and bullying among sexual minority high school students, 2009–2011. J Adolesc Health 2014;55(3):432–8.

22. Pittet I, Berchtold A, Akré C, et al. Are adolescents with chronic conditions particularly at risk for bullying? Arch Dis Child 2010;(9):711–6.

23. Kann L, Kinchen S, Shanklin SL, et al. Youth risk behavior surveillance—United States, 2013. Morbidity and Mortality Weekly Report 2014;63(4):1–68. Surveillance Summaries.

24. Swearer SM, Hymel S. Understanding the psychology of bullying: Moving toward a social-ecological diathesis–stress model. Am Psychol 2015;70(4):344.

25. Young R, Tully M, Ramirez M. School Administrator Perceptions of Cyberbullying Facilitators and Barriers to Preventive Action: A Qualitative Study. Health Educ Behav 2017;44(3):476–84. https://doi.org/10.1177/1090198116673814.

26. Holt MK, Kaufman Kantor G, Finkelhor D. Parent/child concordance about bullying involvement and family characteristics related to bullying and peer victimization. J Sch Violence 2008;8(1):42–63.

27. Zych I, Farrington DP, Ttofi MM. Protective factors against bullying and cyberbullying: A systematic review of meta-analyses. Aggress Violent Behav 2019;45:4–19.

28. Echols L. Social consequences of academic teaming in middle school: The influence of shared course taking on peer victimization. J Educ Psychol 2015;107(1):272.

29. Vitoroulis I, Vaillancourt T. Meta-analytic results of ethnic group differences in peer victimization. Aggress Behav 2015;41(2):149–70.

30. UNESCO. Behind the numbers: Ending school violence and bullying. Available at: https://unesdoc.unesco.org/ark:/48223/pf0000366483. Accessed on February 24, 2023.

31. McDougall P, Vaillancourt T. Long-term adult outcomes of peer victimization in childhood and adolescence: Pathways to adjustment and maladjustment. Am Psychol 2015;70(4):300.

32. Gini G, Pozzoli T. Association between bullying and psychosomatic problems: A meta-analysis. Pediatrics 2009;123(3):1059–65.

33. Lereya ST, Copeland WE, Costello EJ, et al. Adult mental health consequences of peer bullying and maltreatment in childhood: two cohorts in two countries. Lancet Psychiatr 2015;2(6):524–31.

34. Reijntjes A, Kamphuis JH, Prinzie P, et al. Peer victimization and internalizing problems in children: A meta-analysis of longitudinal studies. Child Abuse & Neglect 2010;34(4):244–52.
35. Ttofi MM, Farrington DP, Lösel F, et al. Do the victims of school bullies tend to become depressed later in life? A systematic review and meta-analysis of longitudinal studies. J Aggress Confl Peace Res 2011;3(2):63–73.
36. Bogart LM, Elliott MN, Klein DJ, et al. Peer victimization in fifth grade and health in tenth grade. Pediatrics 2014;133(3):440–7.
37. Armitage R. Bullying in children: impact on child health. BMJ Paediatrics Open 2021;5:e000939. https://doi.org/10.1136/bmjpo-2020-000939.
38. Zarate-Garza PP, Biggs BK, Croarkin P, et al. How Well Do We Understand the Long-Term Health Implications of Childhood Bullying? Harv Rev Psychiatry 2017;25(2):89–95. https://doi.org/10.1097/HRP.0000000000000137.
39. Hawker DS, Boulton MJ. Twenty years' research on peer victimization and psychosocial maladjustment: A meta-analytic review of cross-sectional studies. J Child Psychol Psychiatry Allied Discip 2000;41(4):441–55.
40. Kidger J, Heron J, Leon DA, et al. Self-reported school experience as a predictor of self-harm during adolescence: A prospective cohort study in the South West of England (ALSPAC). J Affect Disord 2015;173:163–9.
41. Klomek AB, Sourander A, Elonheimo H. Bullying by peers in childhood and effects on psychopathology, suicidality, and criminality in adulthood. Lancet Psychiatr 2015;2(10):930–41.
42. Juvonen J, Graham S. Bullying in schools: The power of bullies and the plight of victims. Annu Rev Psychol 2014;65:159–85.
43. Cook CR, Williams KR, Guerra NG, et al. Predictors of bullying and victimization in childhood and adolescence: A meta-analytic investigation. Sch Psychol Q 2010; 25(2):65.
44. Holt MK, Vivolo-Kantor AM, Polanin JR, et al. Bullying and suicidal ideation and behaviors: A meta-analysis. Pediatrics 2015;135(2):e496–509.
45. Kennedy RS. Bully-Victims: An Analysis of Subtypes and Risk Characteristics. J Interpers Violence 2021;36(11–12):5401–21. https://doi.org/10.1177/088626 0517741213.
46. Vaillancourt T, Faris R, Mishna F. Cyberbullying in Children and Youth: Implications for Health and Clinical Practice. Can J Psychiatr 2017;62(6):368–73. https://doi.org/10.1177/0706743716684791.
47. Kerr DCR, Gini G, Capaldi DM. Young men's suicidal behavior, depression, crime, and substance use risks linked to childhood teasing. Child Abuse Negl 2017;67:32–43. https://doi.org/10.1016/j.chiabu.2017.02.026.
48. McGee TR, Scott JG, McGrath JJ, et al. Young adult problem behaviour outcomes of adolescent bullying. J Aggress Confl Peace Res 2011;3(2):110–4.
49. Reijntjes A, Kamphuis JH, Prinzie P, et al. Prospective linkages between peer victimization and externalizing problems in children: A meta-analysis. Aggress Behav 2011;37(3):215–22.
50. Sourander A, Brunstein Klomek A, Kumpulainen K, et al. Bullying at age eight and criminality in adulthood: Findings from the Finnish Nationwide 1981 Birth Cohort Study. Soc Psychiatr Psychiatr Epidemiol 2011;46:1211–9.
51. Reijntjes A, Vermande M, Goossens FA, et al. Developmental trajectories of bullying and social dominance in youth. Child Abuse & Neglect 2013;37(4): 224–34.
52. Flannery DJ, Fox JA, Wallace L, et al. Guns, school shooters, and school safety: What we know and directions for change. Sch Psychol Rev 2021;50(2–3):237–53.

53. Langman P. School Threat Assessments: Psychological and Behavioral Considerations. Journal of Health Service Psychology 2017;43:32–40.

54. Flannery DJ, Modzeleski W, Kretschmar JM. Violence and school shootings. Curr Psychiatr Rep 2013;15:1–7.

55. Flannery DJ, Bear G, Benbenishty R, et al. The scientific evidence supporting an eight point public health oriented action plan to prevent gun violence. In: Osher D, Mayer MJ, Jagers RJ, et al, editors. Keeping students safe and helping them thrive: a collaborative handbook on school safety, mental health, and wellness, II 2019;. p. 227–55.

56. Modzeleski W, Randazzo MR. School threat assessment in the USA: Lessons learned from 15 years of teaching and using the federal model to prevent school shootings. Contemporary School Psychology 2018;22:109–15.

57. Bradshaw CP. Translating research to practice in bullying prevention. Am Psychol 2015;70(4):322.

58. Jiménez-Barbero JA, Ruiz-Hernández JA, Llor-Zaragoza L, et al. Effectiveness of anti-bullying school programs: A meta-analysis. Child Youth Serv Rev 2016;61: 165–75.

59. Johander E, Turunen T, Garandeau CF, et al. Different approaches to address bullying in KiVa schools: Adherence to guidelines, strategies implemented, and outcomes obtained. Prev Sci 2021;22:299–310.

60. Bradshaw CP, Waasdorp TE. Measuring and changing a "culture of bullying". Sch Psychol Rev 2009;38(3):356–61.

61. Ross SW, Horner RH. Bully prevention in positive behavior support. J Appl Behav Anal 2009;42(4):747–59.

62. Farrington DP, Ttofi MM. School-based programs to reduce bullying and victimization. Campbell Systematic Reviews 2009;5(1):i–148.

63. Frey KS, Hirschstein MK, Snell JL, et al. Reducing playground bullying and supporting beliefs: an experimental trial of the steps to respect program. Dev Psychol 2005;41(3):479.

64. Olweus D. Bullying at school: what we know and what we can do (understanding children's worlds). Oxford: Blackwell Publishing; 1993.

65. Gaffney H, Farrington DP. Cyberbullying in the United Kingdom and Ireland. International perspectives on cyberbullying: Prevalence, Risk Factors and Interventions. 2018:101-143.

66. Kennedy RS. A meta-analysis of the outcomes of bullying prevention programs on subtypes of traditional bullying victimization: Verbal, relational, and physical. Aggress Violent Behav 2020;55:101485.

67. Yeager DS, Fong CJ, Lee HY, et al. Declines in efficacy of anti-bullying programs among older adolescents: Theory and a three-level meta-analysis. J Appl Dev Psychol 2015;37:36–51.

68. Lindstrom Johnson S, Waasdorp TE, Gaias LM, et al. Parental responses to bullying: Understanding the role of school policies and practices. J Educ Psychol 2019;(3):475.

69. Waasdorp TE, Bradshaw CP, Duong J. The link between parents' perceptions of the school and their responses to school bullying: Variation by child characteristics and the forms of victimization. J Educ Psychol 2011;103(2):324.

70. Minton SJ. Prejudice and effective anti-bullying intervention: Evidence from the bullying of "minorities". Nord Psychol 2014;66(2):108–20.

71. Bradshaw CP, O'Brennan LM, Waasdorp TE, et al. The new frontier: Leveraging innovative technologies to prevent bullying. In: Vazsonyi AT, Flannery DJ,

DeLisi M, editors. The cambridge handbook of violent behavior and aggression. Cambridge University Press; 2018. p. 635–724.

72. Gini G, Pozzoli T. Bullied children and psychosomatic problems: a meta-analysis. Pediatrics 2013;132(4):720–9.

73. Glew G, Rivara F, Feudtner C. Bullying: children hurting children. Pediatr Rev 2000;21(6):183–9 ; quiz 190.

74. Waseem M, Paul A, Schwartz G, et al. Role of pediatric emergency physicians in identifying bullying. J Emerg Med 2017;52(2):246–52.

75. Shaw JS, Hagan JF, Shepard MT, et al, editors. Bright futures tool and resource kit. 2nd edition. American Academy of Pediatrics; 2019.

76. stopbullying.gov. U.S. Department of Health and Human Services. http://www. stopbullying.gov. Accessed on February 20, 2023.

77. Dickson DJ, Laursen B, Valdes O, et al. Derisive Parenting Fosters Dysregulated Anger in Adolescent Children and Subsequent Difficulties with Peers. J Youth Adolesc 2019;48(8):1567–79.

78. Sausen KA, Randolph JW, Casciato AN, et al. The Development, Preliminary Validation, and Clinical Application of the Quick Parenting Assessment. Prev Sci 2022;23(2):306–20.

A Developmentally Informed Approach to Address Mass Firearm Violence

Ashley Sward, PsyD[a],*, Jodi Zik, MD[a,b],
Amber R. McDonald, PhD, LCSW[a], Laurel Niep, LCSW[a],
Steven Berkowitz, MD[a,b]

KEYWORDS

- Gun violence • Mass shooting • Child • Adolescent • Caregiver
- Pediatric medical provider • Development

KEY POINTS

- Although mass firearm violence is a small subset of gun violence, the psychological effects on children and adolescents are widespread.
- Tools used in response to mass firearm violence are applicable to other forms of community violence.
- The role of the pediatric provider is to engage caregivers to respond to the child appropriately and effectively in the aftermath of mass firearm violence. Tools to support caregivers include modeling appropriate response in clinic, highlighting developmental considerations, and providing appropriate education materials.
- Pediatric providers should be aware of symptoms of secondary trauma and burnout. Reflection on and support of provider's well-being is strongly encouraged.

INTRODUCTION

Although mass gun violence has become a regular headline in the media, there is a lack of agreement regarding its exact definition. Some define a "mass violence event" as one in which 3 or more victims are killed in one location within one event[1]; the Federal Bureau of Investigation (FBI) requires 4 or more casualties, excluding the perpetrator, and still others use the definition of 4 or more individuals with fatal or nonfatal injuries from one event.[2] From a psychological perspective, any violent event resulting in numerable fatalities or injuries would qualify. Although most pediatricians will not

[a] Department of Psychiatry, University of Colorado School of Medicine, Anschutz Medical Campus, 1890 North Revere Court, Suite 4092, Aurora, CO 80045, USA; [b] Department of Pediatrics, University of Colorado School of Medicine, Anschutz Medical Campus, 1890 North Revere Court, Suite 4092, Aurora, CO 80045, USA
* Corresponding author.
E-mail address: ashley.sward@cuanschutz.edu

Pediatr Clin N Am 70 (2023) 1171–1182
https://doi.org/10.1016/j.pcl.2023.06.009
0031-3955/23/© 2023 Elsevier Inc. All rights reserved.

provide direct care for a physical injury as a result from a mass shooting, the secondary trauma from such events undoubtably permeates pediatric offices across the country. Social media platforms amplify the trauma and grief of communities impacted by these horrific events, which contributes to the increased anxiety and depression among our youth treated by pediatricians.[3–5]

Considerations regarding gun violence in general have become a necessity in pediatric practice. According to data from the Centers for Disease Control and Prevention from 2016 to 2020, more than 3500 children and teens (0–19) were shot and killed in America and another 15,000 were wounded in shootings. Of those deaths, 2100 are homicides (often domestic violence or street violence), 1200 are suicide by gun, 130 are unintentional shootings, and 25 or fewer are the result of mass shootings.[6] The *Gun Violence Archive* noted 648 mass shootings in 2022 alone, 66 of which meet Burgess' criteria for mass violence,[1] and 38 of which meet FBI criteria.[2] Although precise numbers are unclear, gun violence in general was the leading cause of death for children and teens in 2020, and the devastation left in its wake has become very clear.

Although mass shootings are only a small subset of gun violence events, the psychological effects of mass shootings are widespread in part owing to their high media attention. Mass shootings have extensive and varied impacts on mental health and perceptions of safety regardless of relationship to the violence. One does not have to be present at a violent event to suffer negative effects. Media exposure can lead to significant anxiety, fears, and impairment, sometimes leading to a self-perpetuating cycle of fear and media consumption.[7,8] Over the last several years, fear of mass shootings only increased. Many teenagers express worries about shootings happening at their school.[9,10]

School shootings are an even smaller subset of gun violence events that receive significant public attention. Despite being rare, these attacks are incredibly catalyzing and polarizing events. After the Sandy Hook shooting in December 2012, then-President Obama formed a special investigative committee leading to 23 gun violence reduction executive actions. Gun safety legislation is consistently a topic of local and national political debate. Active shooter drills now take place alongside fire drills in American schools for every grade. Since the Austin Tower shootings at the University of Texas, both school and community shootings are increasing significantly and at a greater rate each year.[11] Moreover, victims of school shootings are trending younger. In fact, during the 2020–2021 academic year, more shootings took place in elementary schools than in high schools.[12] Such escalating trends in school and community mass violence simultaneously result in an increase of exposure, both directly and indirectly, for children across the age and developmental spans.

THE ROLE OF PEDIATRICIANS

In response to a mass violence tragedy, and community violence in general, children need access to reliable, supportive adults to help them manage their feelings, organize their thoughts, and monitor for concerning symptoms. Outside of caregivers and teachers, pediatricians have some of the most frequent, consistent contact with children and families from all demographics. Thus, the role of the pediatric provider is vital in addressing community violence, and in particular, mass shooting violence. However, the pediatric provider's time is limited and best used by modeling and providing developmentally grounded guidance to the caregiver, who can then engage with the child on an on-going basis. In engaging the caregiver, the pediatric provider extends the reach of their intervention beyond the office and further promotes the caregiver-child relationship.

A FLEXIBLE FRAMEWORK

It is unlikely that one approach, one manual, or one toolkit is sufficient to meet the needs and constraints of all pediatric providers. As such, the authors reviewed extant literature from key fields about the important aspects of response to a mass shooting. They offer a flexible framework for pediatric providers and include specific age-related suggestions. The prevailing recommendations of the mental health and pediatric fields are as follows: (1) to engage in intentional, direct, and age-appropriate conversations about the facts of the event; (2) to create space for children to share their emotions and experiences; (3) to provide reliable structure and routine; (4) to encourage healthy and effective coping; and (5) to assess for posttraumatic stress (PTS) symptoms and refer for intervention as needed.[13–17]

Engage in Intentional, Direct, and Age-Appropriate Conversations in the Direct Aftermath of a Traumatic Event

Engaging children in conversation and asking them about their perception or knowledge of events is critical to initiating an open dialogue, and for adults to understand what children already know, including what accurate or inaccurate information is formulating their response. It is recommended that adults follow the child's lead during the conversation—asking what questions the child has, responding to questions that are asked, and sharing the information needed without extra emotional or graphic detail. The American Academy of Pediatrics (AAP) notes that adults should keep the conversation straightforward and direct, providing basic information and being clear even with young children.[18] If adults share more information than the child is able to process given their age and development, it is likely to cause confusion or additional harm. This recommendation points to the importance of considering the age and development of the child when responding and sharing information. When children feel they are not getting their questions answered or that the adults are not comfortable discussing these difficult topics, they are likely to look for answers from less reliable sources, such as social media or less filtered sources, such as repeat media coverage, including graphic scenes and emotional interviews.

To support the caregiver of an infant or young child, it is important to remember that many adults continue to believe that very young children are not as impacted by tragedy as older children, assuming that the child is too young to notice. More specific guidance and rationale may be required for caregivers of young children given these misperceptions. Often it is sufficient to tell the younger child that we (the caregivers) make sure they are safe. Highlighting the importance of the caregiver's role in buffering the child from stress can help increase a caregiver's confidence in responding to their young child. When supporting the caregiver of an elementary or middle school–aged child, the pediatric provider should be aware of misinformation about retraumatization. If a child does not initiate a conversation in the aftermath of a traumatic experience, adults often feel relief and assume it is for the best if tough conversations do not arise. They may worry that talking directly to the child about their experience will create more stress. However, we know that a caregiver's ability to recognize and initiate the discussion with the child at their developmental level is protective and can ameliorate stress—encouraging the child to rely on their caregiver for information rather than to use less trustworthy sources. Although this is true of teenagers as well, it is even more likely that by the time the caregiver initiates the conversation, the teen has already been exposed to a great deal of outside influence. Moreover, most teens are in a second stage of developmental independence, which may make them less willing to engage in these conversations. Parents should be reassured to respect the wishes of a teen without colluding with avoidance. Pediatricians can encourage the caregiver to share some of their own thoughts, feelings, and reactions to reinforce open communication and connection. Another approach is to ask one's teen what their friends are saying about the event. Often, they will tell their own thoughts and feelings in the process.

Create Space for Children to Share Their Emotions and Experience over Time

In the aftermath of direct or indirect exposure to mass gun violence, most children are likely to continue to approach trusted adults to process their experiences and emotions even after the facts of the event are established. During these conversations, it is recommended that adults encourage children to express their feelings and provide consistent validation of the child's emotional experience. It is important for children to know that it is normative and OK to feel strong emotions associated with the traumatic event. However, it is also important to separate the validation of a child's emotions from reinforcement of inaccurate or unhelpful thoughts. The pediatrician's role includes anticipating common feelings and reactions based on the child's developmental level and encouraging the caregiver to hold a safe space for the child to share their story, process their emotions, and get gentle, corrective feedback.

A child's age and developmental level are particularly important aspects in how they experience and respond to traumatic events. For example, very young children often feel a challenging combination of responsibility and helplessness in the wake of traumatic exposure. This makes sense given that they are in the preoperational stage of cognitive development characterized by egocentrism and centration. In addition, infants and young children are much more likely to express reactions and emotions physically and behaviorally given limited language ability. This may present as the loss of previously gained developmental skills, changes in relational patterns, or traumatic play. Traumatic play is characterized by repetitive behaviors and less imaginative themes often tied to a child's continued focus on aspects or attempts to change the outcome of a traumatic event. The Child Mind Institute notes the importance of play for processing in young children and encourages adults to keep an eye out for opportunities to encourage nurturing and security themes when appropriate.[19] School-aged children are likely to respond by expressing fear about their own safety and the safety of loved ones, as well as guilt if they have a direct connection to the event. Although they are also at risk for developmental regression, their stress is more likely to translate physically as somatic complaints, sleep disruption, and difficulties with concentration and focus.[20] School-aged children have more ability than their younger peers to share their reactions and feelings with others. Pediatricians should encourage caregivers to have conversations with their child exploring when and with whom they should discuss their experience. Adolescents and teens often require more encouragement to open up to their caregivers about their feelings. Their feelings are likely to include guilt, shame, and vulnerability. Managing feelings of embarrassment about their response to the mass violence may necessitate direct guidance from the pediatrician to the child. It is also not uncommon for teens to be angry in response to a mass shooting. Fantasies of revenge should be acknowledged with validation for the underlying feeling and include gentle redirection toward more constructive action (advocacy, art, and so forth).

Provide Reliable Structure and Routine

In the midst of the emotional and often physical chaos that mass violence leaves in its wake, the importance of maintaining safety and routine at home cannot be understated, as this provides a sense of security while children try to make sense of violent events. Fueled by feelings of guilt and concerns that too much is being asked of the child, caregivers may become overly permissive in response to a child's exposure to a traumatic event. It is important for the pediatrician to address this upon recognition of such patterns or bring it up in the context of anticipatory guidance. Moreover, caregivers may need more specific guidance about expectations for structure and routine. There are 3 key ingredients in creating structure for children: consistency, predictability, and follow-through.[21] The day-to-day implementation and how much the caregiver may need to support these features depend on the age and developmental level of the child but largely follows the general developmental guidance typically presented to different age groups unaffected by trauma exposure. Structure for children relies heavily on the consistency, predictability, and follow-through of parental response. Caregivers of children of all ages benefit from counseling around the importance of maintaining the consistency of expectations, predictability of limits, and follow-through on consequences while maintaining empathy for what the child has experienced. Very young children need significant caregiver support to establish and maintain routines especially if the mass violence exposure has impacted the child's sleeping, eating, and/or soothing. Moreover, repeated interaction of a young child expressing a need, and the need being consistently met by the caregiver, is the basis for attachment security and buffering in the face of adversity. School-aged children are likely to have increased consistency, predictability, and follow-through inherently provided by school and extracurricular activities. However, caregivers of school-aged children often require support and guidance to ensure such structure is maintained in the face of a traumatic event, particularly if it involves school or other community supports. Note that older children are more likely to push boundaries to test parental response and their own sense of safety. Teenagers are especially likely to rebel against rules and structure. Although this is developmentally normative, new rebellious activities in the wake of a traumatic event or shooting should be met with the same consistency of expectations, predictability of limits, and follow-through on consequences to model safety and routine.

Encourage Healthy and Effective Coping

Healthy and effective coping strategies should instill a sense of calm, efficacy, and connection to children and families in response to a mass violence event. Teaching and encouraging age-appropriate relaxation and mindfulness skills can support the increase of children's sense of calm. Preschoolers may enjoy tensing and relaxing their bodies like "dry and cooked spaghetti." Elementary school-aged children and preadolescents may benefit from a relaxation script or application featuring their favorite TV show character, whereas teenagers may be able to find calm and solace by hiking outdoors. Different relaxing activities and outlets are important for the pediatrician to explore with children of all ages and their families. Moreover, reminding caregivers of the importance of offering consistent reassurance of the child's safety in the aftermath of trauma is encouraged. Helplessness is a common feeling in response to mass gun violence at any age. Increasing a sense of efficacy can help address feelings of helplessness in the aftermath. Helping a young child regain a developmental skill lost to traumatic exposure increases their sense of efficacy, confidence, and control. As children progress in age, they may benefit from opportunities to increase their sense of efficacy in relation to the traumatic event. Engaging in advocacy opportunities and exploring the constructive things they did during the shooting to support their or others' safety are some examples. Memorials and vigils are commonplace in response to mass violence events. Although such events may be a good opportunity for older children to offer and receive support from peers and community members, special consideration to the timing, level of attention to victims and perpetrators, and developmental suitability of content is encouraged. One of the greatest protective factors in any traumatic exposure for a child is having at least one safe, responsive caregiver who can provide a buffering effect to traumatic stress. The importance of caregiver engagement is not groundbreaking news in pediatrics. The adverse childhood experiences (ACE) study and subsequent advances in developmental and toxic stress research ushered in a new understanding of the role of the caregiver in mediating traumatic stress. It emphasized the importance of relationships for optimal child development as well as long-term behavioral and physical health outcomes. The National Child Traumatic Stress Network (NCTSN) and US Department of Education highlight the importance of maintaining and increasing connection for children—with family, friends, and community. The pediatrician should engage caregivers in monitoring their child's relationship patterns after a mass shooting. Desire to withdraw, irritability, and anxiety in public places are just a few common reactions to mass shootings that can impact a child's connection with others. Last, the evidence is sound that repeat media coverage, including graphic scenes, sensationalized coverage, and emotional interviews, is detrimental to children. For this reason, another shared recommendation is to limit children's access to media coverage. For older children, the AAP recommends that caregivers record media coverage and watch it themselves before viewing with children in order to be prepared to support them in processing what they see and hear. Older children and teens are also more likely to have immediate, uninterrupted access to media coverage via their cell phones and social media. The AAP recommends that caregivers be aware of what information exists and take steps to proactively speak with their children about what they are likely to see and hear. Families can also set guidelines to support children in limiting their media consumption—removing certain apps or silencing notifications for a period of time, setting time limits for how long they watch news coverage, and opening channels of communication to discuss content children observe and how they respond to that information. The AAP Council on Communications and Media has also created tools such as the Family Media Use Plan to support families in identifying limits and boundaries for media consumption.[22]

Assess for Psychiatric Symptoms and Refer for Intervention as Needed

Not all children are impacted to the same extent by exposure to similar traumatic events. However, it is imperative for the pediatric provider to assess for posttraumatic stress reactions in the aftermath of a mass violence event, as early identification and early intervention promise to limit long-term impairment. PTS is a set of psychological and physiologic responses that children may experience in the aftermath of a traumatic event. These responses include reexperiencing, avoidance, and hyperarousal, as well as changes in thinking and mood. When these responses persist between 3 and 30 days and cause impairment, the child meets criteria for Acute Stress Disorder. When these responses last beyond 30 days and cause impairment, the child meets criteria for posttraumatic stress disorder (PTSD). The goal of immediate response in the wake of trauma is to identify and address PTS responses early so the child avoids developing PTSD diagnosis and associated impairment. Trauma screening in pediatrics is highly recommended as a general practice. NCTSN described trauma screening as a brief, focused tool or process used to determine exposure, reaction, and subsequent mental health needs related to a traumatic event and is considered a "wide net" process for identification. There are multiple assessment and screening tools that assist providers in identifying symptoms of PTS (Table 1). However, it is important to balance the burden of the screening measure with the importance of information

Table 1 Posttraumatic Stress Symptom Screening Tools		
Age Range	**Tool**	**Description**
9 mo to 6 y	Diagnostic Infant and Preschool Assessment (DIPA)	The DIPA is a structured caregiver interview with 13 self-contained modules linked to *Diagnostic and Statistical Manual of Mental Disorders* (*DSM*) criteria, one of which includes PTSD
3 to17 y	The Child and Adolescent Trauma Screen (CATS)	The CATS is a widely accessible screener measuring exposure and reactions based on *DSM-5* criteria for PTSD. It includes a self-report for ages 7–17 and 2 versions of a caregiver report for ages 3–6 and 7–17
0 to 19 y	The PEdiatric ACEs and Related Life-events Screener (PEARLS)	PEARLS screens for a child's exposure to ACEs. It includes a self-report for ages 12-19 and 2 versions of a caregiver: reports for ages 0-11 and 12-19. It does not include symptom measure

it can provide in a timely manner. As such, a targeted approach to screening in response to a mass shooting is recommended. Established risk factors, including physical proximity to the place of the shooting, close personal connection to those directly exposed, and overlapping identities with targeted individuals or groups, should prompt the pediatric provider to assess further for PTS. Other risk factors of general trauma include previous experience of death or injury to a loved one, history of depression, anxiety or other mood concerns, and previous trauma exposure. Further assessment of PTS without the use of a screening measure requires the pediatric provider to familiarize themselves with the criteria for the various PTS responses and how those responses present according to the child's age and developmental level.

Similar to recommendations around other physical and behavioral health screening and assessment processes, it is imperative to identify recommendations and referrals before implementation. When a child is identified as meeting criteria for Acute Stress Disorder, PTSD, or related diagnoses (ie, Depression, Anxiety), or is likely to develop a disorder without intervention, the pediatric provider must know where or to whom to refer for follow-up. This may be one of the most challenging aspects of care owing to a significant lack of mental health funding and resources across the country. Although the importance of pediatric mental health services is increasingly recognized, the need continues to far exceed the capacity. This is particularly true in rural areas, as well as for black, indigenous, and people of color who face significant access disparities. If the pediatric provider is fortunate to have access to a community resource or behavioral health navigator, there is greater support to ensure children and families connect to needed interventions and treatment. Nearly as important as the identification of a reputable, accessible, and available treatment provider is the ability of the care navigator to facilitate a "warm handoff" to increase likelihood of engagement in recommended services.

Although not available in all clinics, integrated behavioral health (IBH) in pediatrics is a significant resource to support children and families in the aftermath of a mass shooting. Pediatricians are limited in their scope to intervene by time constraints, billing requirements, and training focus. Close collaboration with an IBH provider increases the child and families' connection to universal, targeted, and/or intensive support as identified by either the pediatric or the IBH provider. In the absence of IBH access, many pediatricians have access to a child psychiatry access program (CPAP). Such programs are designed to immediately connect pediatric providers to mental health consultation to aid in the diagnostic assessment, treatment recommendations, and resource needs of patients. The National Network of Child Psychiatry Programs, established in 2011, is a national organization supporting new and existing CPAP programs throughout the country (https://www.nncpap.org/). Currently, there are established or Health Resources and Services Administration-funded CPAP programs in all but 4 states in the United States.

BEYOND RESPONSE

Although vital, a pediatrician's direct clinical screening and support of children and families in the aftermath of a mass shooting is only a piece of their role. As previously mentioned, mass gun violence is a small subset of America's gun violence epidemic. In 2020, firearms became the leading cause of death for children and adolescents, surpassing motor vehicle and other accidental injuries.[23] Proactively addressing mass gun violence requires firearm violence prevention strategies. In 2022, the AAP released the *Firearm-Related Injuries and Deaths in Children and Youth: Injury Prevention and Harm Reduction* policy statement and accompanying technical report. The statement urges pediatric providers to adopt a harm-reduction approach with multilayered strategies in their practices and beyond.[24]

Addressing gun violence prevention at a practice level includes anticipatory guidance for mental health screening, lethal means counseling, and safe firearm storage. When discussing mental health screening as a preventive approach to mass gun violence, it is important to clarify that a direct association between mental illness and mass gun violence is not established. Rather, it is one piece of the complex constellation of risk and protective factors associated with gun violence. However, screening and subsequent mental health treatment are tools to identify and intervene with children at higher risk for violence to self or others owing to mental illness, suicidal thoughts, desperation, and/or hopelessness. Lethal means counseling and safe firearm storage include asking older children and all parents about the presence of guns in their homes and advising on separation and locking of ammunition and guns with codes/keys not available to kids. These evidence-based strategies are quick, simple, and powerful ways for pediatricians to influence access to weapons and gun deaths. Addressing gun violence outside of the pediatric office requires engagement in policy and legislation. AAP was founded upon advocacy. It formed after intentional separation from the American Medical Association (AMA) in response to the AMA's refusal to endorse legislation supporting maternal and child health initiatives. Advocacy is now a Common Program Requirement in pediatric residency training. Statements released by the AAP, Pediatric Trauma Society, and American College of Surgeons strongly encourage members to take action to address firearm safety in the form of advocacy.

Advocacy efforts with the strongest evidence base to impact gun violence include increased funding for firearm violence prevention research and programming, and increased regulation of the availability, design, and storage of firearms.[23] Research for gun violence prevention is a vital resource. In response to the Dickey amendment in 1996 prohibiting federal funding for gun violence research, there are significant gaps in gun violence information that need to be addressed.[25] Funding for the identification and dissemination of evidence-informed, community-based violence intervention programs is also needed. Stronger, more effective gun legislation should be enacted and enforced at state and national levels.

The single most effective measure to reduce firearm injury and death is the absence of guns in homes and communities. Legislation to target universal background checks, safe storage of firearms, extreme risk protection orders (also known as red flag laws), and assault-style weapons bans are other evidence-based methods of gun violence prevention to be supported by pediatricians.[26] Last, regulation of safety measures, such as licensing, training, registration, and insurance, much like other consumer products should be considered. It is important to note that when evidence-based measures are not demanded at local, state, and national levels, poorly researched and planned measures are enacted and can have deleterious effects. According to a National Center for Education Statistics study conducted during the 2015–2016 school year, 95% of public schools performed an active shooter drill.[27] The effectiveness of such drills to prevention of injury and death is unclear, but preliminary findings show compelling evidence of psychological harm to students.[28]

SELF-CARE

Crucial to the pediatrician's roles in the prevention and response to mass shootings is self-care. Burnout rates for health care workers continue to rise. Demanding clinical work; frequent exposure to sickness, trauma, injury, and death; long hours; and ever-increasing expectations pave the way for compassion fatigue and burnout. Burnout and compassion fatigue are even more likely when dealing with a mass shooting. As a member of a community impacted by a mass shooting, the pediatric provider may have personal connections that require attention and support. Although burnout has received increased attention in the past several years, effective, sustainable strategies have been slow to follow. One recent nationwide study of physicians found balanced nutrition, strong friendships, and peer support were the strongest protective factors against burnout. Peer support combined with professional coaching was particularly protective. Collaboration with mental health professionals trained to address burnout and compassion fatigue is a recent phenomenon gaining traction and evidence. This may present another good opportunity to collaborate with IBH providers. Integrated mental health professionals are in a good position to support pediatric providers through training and consultative support in the areas of vicarious trauma, burnout, and compassion fatigue. It is important to acknowledge that many of these strategies are considered the responsibility of the individual rather than the system. Health care organizations must begin to reconcile that such stress-related injuries are inherent risks to the provider's role and increase systemic support. Of note, the military has pioneered several organizational approaches to address role-related stress injuries. The stress continuum model was initially developed by the US Marines.[29] It is a tool that, when adapted to other settings such as health care, can promote shared language and conceptual agreement of stress states throughout the system with the goal of decreasing stigma and increasing varying levels of organizational support.

SUMMARY

Although mass shooting events account for a small subset of gun violence in America, they continue to increase at an alarming rate and have far-reaching psychological impact on children and adolescents. Pediatric providers must be ready to provide developmentally appropriate responses in the aftermath of such tragedy. Common recommendations culled from the behavioral health and pediatric fields include the following: engaging in intentional, direct, and age-appropriate conversations; creating space for children to share their emotions and experiences; maintaining structure and routine; encouraging healthy and effective coping; and assessing for and responding to PTS symptoms.[13–17] Pediatricians are encouraged to use modeling and caregiver engagement to support these responses to children of varying ages and stages of development. Although support for children and families in the aftermath of a mass gun violence event is important, strategies must also be considered from a preventive standpoint. Pediatric providers are encouraged to adopt harm reduction approaches to gun violence during regular pediatric visits and become active in advocacy efforts to help address America's gun violence epidemic.

CLINICS CARE POINTS

- Confirm the child's developmental level is commensurate with chronologic age and adjust guidance as needed.

- Modeling to a caregiver how to start a difficult, developmentally appropriate conversation with their child is an effective way to guide and educate them during a visit.

- Encouraging and equipping caregivers to be the direct source of developmentally grounded, factual information about a traumatic event may dissuade children from seeking information from less reputable and/or more sensationalized sources.

- Caregivers often need additional guidance and encouragement to maintain consistency and predictability and to follow through routines, expectations, and limits in the aftermath of trauma exposure.

- In terms of prevention of mass firearm tragedies, advocacy is encouraged, and it should be kept in mind that the single most effective measure to reduce firearm injury and death is the absence of guns in homes and communities.

DISCLOSURE

There are no financial conflicts of interest to disclose.

REFERENCES

1. Burgess AW. Mass, spree and serial homicide. In: Douglas J, Burgess AW, Burgess AG, et al, editors. Crime classification manual. 2nd Edition. San Francisco, CA: Jossey Bass; 2006. p. 437–70.
2. Mass Shooting Methodology and Reasoning. In: Gun Violence Archive. Available at: https://www.gunviolencearchive.org/. Updated October 25, 2022. Accessed October 27, 2022.
3. Pyrooz D, Moule, RJ. Gangs and social media. In: Oxford Research Encyclopedia of Criminology. Available at: https://oxfordre.com/criminology/view/10.1093/acrefore/9780190264079.001.0001/acrefore-9780190264079-e-439. Accessed February 27, 2023.
4. Lane J. The digital street. New York NY: Oxford University Press; 2018.
5. Crouch JL, Hanson RF, Saunders BE, et al. Income, race/ethnicity, and exposure to violence in youth: Results from the national survey of adolescents. J Community Psychol 2000;28(6):625–41.
6. The impact of gun violence on children and teens fact sheet. In: Everytown Research and Policy. Available at: https://everytownresearch.org/report/the-

impact-of-gun-violence-on-children-and-teens/#key-findings. May 29, 2019. Accessed October 25, 2022.

7. Thompson RR, Jones NM, Holman EA, et al. Media exposure to mass violence events can fuel a cycle of distress. Sci Adv 2019;5(4):3502.

8. Riehm KE, Adams LB, Krueger EA, et al. Adolescents' concerns about school violence or shootings and association with depressive, anxiety, and panic symptoms. JAMA Netw Open 2021;4(11):e2132131.

9. Colin O, Kanako T. Alpha and beta changes in anxiety in response to mass shooting related information. Pers Indiv Differ 2022;186(A):e111326.

10. Graff N. Stress of mass shootings causing cascade of collective traumas. In: Monitor on Psychology. Available at: https://www.apa.org/monitor/2022/09/news-mass-shootings-collective-traumas?amp%3Bamp%3Bamp. Published April 18, 2018. Accessed October 27, 2022.

11. Schultz JM, Cohen AM, Muschert GW. Fatal school shootings and the epidemiological context of firearm mortality in the United States. Disaster Health 2013;1(2): 84–101.

12. National Center for Education Statistics analyzing data. In: Homeland Defense and Security. Available at: https://www.chds.us/ssdb/. Accessed January 26, 2023.

13. Schonfield DJ, Demaria T. Providing psychosocial support to children and families in the aftermath of disasters and crises. Pediatrics 2015;136(4):1120–30.

14. Talking to children about violence: tips for parents and teachers. National Association of School Psychologists. Available at: https://www.nasponline.org/resources-and-publications/resources-and-podcasts/school-safety-and-crisis/school-violence-resources/talking-to-children-about-violence-tips-for-parents-and-teachers. Accessed October 6, 2022.

15. Helping your children manage distress in the aftermath of a shooting. In: American Psychological Association. Available at: https://www.apa.org/topics/gun-violence-crime/shooting-aftermath. February 1, 2019. Accessed October 6, 2022.

16. Talking to children about the shooting. In: National Child Traumatic Stress Network Tip Sheet. Available at: https://www.nctsn.org/resources/talking-children-about-shooting. Published in 2014. Accessed October 6, 2022.

17. Tips for talking with and helping children and youth cope after a disaster or traumatic event: A guide for parents, caregivers, and teachers. In: Substance Abuse and Mental Health Service Administration Tip Sheet. Available at: https://store.samhsa.gov/sites/default/files/d7/priv/sma12-4732.pdf. Revised 2013. Accessed October 7, 2022.

18. Helping children cope and adjust after a disaster. In: Academy of Pediatrics. Available at: https://www.aap.org/en/patient-care/disasters-and-children/disaster-management-resources-by-topic/helping-children-cope-and-adjust-after-a-disaster/. Last Update November 10, 2021. Accessed October 6, 2022.

19. Helping children cope after a traumatic event. In: Child Mind Institute. Available at: https://childmind.org/guide/helping-children-cope-after-a-traumatic-event.pdf. Updated February 23, 2023. Accessed February 27, 2023.

20. Age-related reactions to a traumatic event. In: National Child Traumatic Stress Network Tip Sheet. Available at: https://www.nctsn.org/sites/default/files/resources//age_related_reactions_to_traumatic_events.pdf. Accessed January 26, 2023.

21. Building structure. In: Centers for Disease Control and Prevention. Available at: https://www.cdc.gov/parents/essentials/toddlersandpreschoolers/structure/building.html. Reviewed November 5, 2019. Accessed February 25, 2023.

22. American Academy of Pediatrics. Family Media Plan. https://www.healthychildren. org/English/fmp/Pages/MediaPlan.aspx .Accessed April 17, 2023.

23. Goldstick JE, Cunningham RM, Carter PM. Current causes of death in children and adolescents in the United States. N Engl J Med 2022;386(20):1955–6.

24. Lee LK, Fleegler EW, Goyal MK, et al. Firearm-related injuries and deaths in children and youth: injury prevention and harm reduction. Pediatrics 2022;150(6): 60–70.

25. Cost estimate of federal funding for gun violence research and data infrastructure. In: Health Management Associates. Available at: https://assets.joycefdn. org/content/uploads/CostEstimateofFederalFundingforGunViolenceResearch. pdf?mtime=20210712175851&focal=none. Accessed February 25, 2023.

26. Dowd MD, Sege RD, Gardner HG. Firearm-related injuries affecting the pediatric population. Pediatrics 2012;130(5):1416–23.

27. 1. Diliberti M, Jackson M, Kemp J. Crime, violence, discipline, and safety in U.S. public schools: findings from the school survey on crime and safety: 2015-16. US Department of Education, National Center for Education Statistics. Published 2017. Available at: https://nces.ed.gov/pubsearch/pubsinfo.asp?pubid=2019 061. Accessed April 18, 2023.

28. Graf N. A majority of U.S. teens fear a shooting could happen at their school, and most parents share their concern. Pew Research Center. Published April 18, 2018. https://www.pewresearch.org/fact-tank/2018/04/18/a-majority-of-u-s-teens-fear-ashooting-could-happen-at-their-school-and-mostparents-share-their-concern/. Accessed April 18, 2023.

29. Nash W, Krantz L, Stein N, et al. Comprehensive soldier fitness, battle mind, and the stress continuum model: military organizational approaches to prevention. In: Ruzek JI, Schnurr PP, Vasterling JJ, et al, editors. Caring for veterans with deployment-related stress disorders. Washington DC: American Psychological Association; 2011. p. 193–214.

Violence Exposure and Trauma-Informed Care

Michael Arenson, MD, MS, MA[a,b,*], Heather Forkey, MD[a,b,c,d]

KEYWORDS

- Trauma-informed care • Toxic stress • Relational health • Human stress response
- Child development • Adverse childhood experiences
- Positive childhood experiences

KEY POINTS

- Instead of just summing the suffering, help patients and families build the buffering of relational health.
- If you hear about toxic stress-associated symptoms, think about trauma; If you hear about trauma, think about symptoms.
- TIC is the practice that guides pediatricians in helping children experiencing toxic stress while simultaneously promoting relational health and resilience of children.
- In the face of violence concerns, pediatricians should screen for exposures, symptoms, and safety; voice and validate the patient's experience; provide brief interventions in the pediatric setting to address symptoms; and if needed, refer to evidence-based therapies.
- Build webs of support around the child in the community, including family, school, and faith-based settings, and other child-focused programs (eg, Boys and Girls Club).

INTRODUCTION

Addressing violence in pediatrics requires a working knowledge of trauma-informed care (TIC). TIC weaves together our current understanding of evolution, child development, and human physiology and explains common childhood responses to traumatic events. In this article, we describe our current approach to treating childhood trauma in the context of violence.

We begin with how human biology—which has evolved over time to help us survive—can ultimately result in a maladaptive biologic process called toxic stress. Downstream effects of toxic stress are dysfunction at genetic, molecular, organ, and ultimately

[a] UMass Memorial Children's Medical Center, UMass Chan Medical School, 55 Lake Avenue North, Worcester, MA 01655, USA; [b] Center for Child Health Equity; [c] Foster Children Evaluation Service (FaCES); [d] Department of Pediatrics, University of Massachusetts Chan Medical School, Worcester, MA, USA
* Corresponding author.
E-mail address: michael.arenson@umassmed.edu

Pediatr Clin N Am 70 (2023) 1183–1200
https://doi.org/10.1016/j.pcl.2023.06.010

behavioral levels. We will discuss how the pediatrician can identify, diagnose, and treat these consequences.

Ultimately, TIC relies on the pediatrician's ability to keep trauma high on their differential diagnosis. A child naturally builds resilience as a part of their typical development, and TIC is the pediatrician's tool to prevent or address barriers to this natural process. TIC leverages a child's natural strengths and biologic processes by (1) scaffolding the patient's relationships to safe, stable, and nurturing adults and (2) strengthening core skills for resilience (eg, planning, adapting, and achieving goals) while responding to symptoms if necessary.[1]

It is our hope to change the perception that TIC is a trendy topic or one that requires a disruptive change in practice. With some simple modifications in common knowledge and practice, pediatricians will find that TIC blends into their current daily patient care routine without much hassle and may simultaneously make patient care more effective, predictable, and rewarding.

Background

Biologic Foundations of TIC: The human stress response and the buffering effect of safe, stable, and nurturing adult relationships (SSNRs).

Humans have an "appetite" for social connection. In the same way we get hungry when we have not eaten, a biologic signaling system may come into play if one's social relationships fall below an acceptable level. This is likely mediated on the molecular level by the hormone oxytocin, endogenous opioids, and dopaminergic pathways.[2] In addition to signaling a hunger for social connection, research shows that oxytocin also buffers human stress responses.

Thus, in addition to fight–flight–freeze, humans have another stress response, namely "affiliate" or "tend and befriend," in which oxytocin is implicated in the seeking of affiliative contact in response to stress (**Fig. 1**).[3] These 4 stress responses have

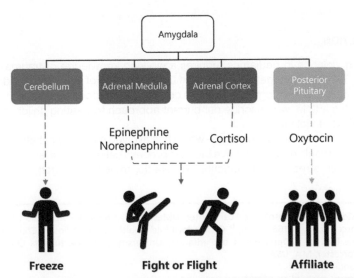

Fig. 1. The 4 major behavioral responses to a threat. (*Adapted from* Garner AS, Saul RA. Defining adversity and toxic stress. In: Thinking Developmentally: Nurturing Wellness in Childhood to Promote Lifelong Health. American Academy of Pediatrics. 2018:13-24; with permission.)

been posited to have a neurobiological hierarchy; when we experience stress, our bodies' preference is to manage it with, "a little help from our friends." That is to say, we create dyadic, mutually regulated systems of stress relief through SSNR.[4] This has an evolutionary advantage—for example, although humans could not fight a bear or lion alone, our unique ability to band together under stress and work toward common goals gives us an advantage. This is the underpinning of why humans need SSNR.

All children experience stress and adversity at some point in life but when it is managed within the context of nurturing relationships, such events can be weathered and even used for growth. When SSNR are unavailable or insufficient, our neurobiological stress response shunts from affiliative to the fight–flight–freeze pathway. A person whose body is in fight–flight–freeze mode experiences a cascade of stress hormones and biological processes in response.[5] If the stress is prolonged, frequent, or severe and there is a marked imbalance between stressors and protective factors, "toxic stress" can result (which we discuss in detail below).[6] Many stressors can cause toxic stress, including violence within a child's family, community, or by an intimate partner in the home. Thus, the toxic stress response results from 2 components: (1) The effect of the adverse event(s) and (2) the insufficiency of protective relationships.

Adverse Childhood Experiences, Violence, and Trauma-Informed Care

Our current understanding of the association of childhood adversity and subsequent health consequences is greatly informed by the Adverse Childhood Experience (ACE) Study.[7] The investigators developed the ACE score, an integer count of 10 adverse experiences during childhood (range, 0–10), which has repeatedly demonstrated a strong, graded, dose–response relationship to numerous health and social outcomes (eg, mental illness, illicit drug use, suicide risk, and risk for chronic diseases) in a variety of populations.[8,9] Rightfully, the ACE study has attracted significant scientific and policy attention.[10] More recently, the ACE score has gained attention through lay press and websites,[11] and the ACE score is increasingly being used and promoted as a clinical screening tool at the individual level.[12]

However, cautions have been raised about using ACE scores as a clinical tool.[9,13–15] ACE scores are a relatively crude measure of cumulative childhood toxic stress exposure that can vary widely from person to person.[16] It has validity as a risk identification tool in populations but not individuals. Unlike true screening measures, such as blood pressure or lipid levels that use measurement reference standards and cutoff points or thresholds for clinical decision-making, the ACE score is neither a standardized measure of childhood exposure to toxic stress nor does it have defined predictive value for later outcomes. Perhaps, most concerning is the suggestion that it inappropriately reduces patients' histories to a number. For example, is, "My father raped me when I was 5 years old," reliably and meaningfully reduced to an ACE score of "1"? Alternatively, is being physically beaten once the same as being beaten weekly for years, and do they both deserve an ACE score of "1"?

Nevertheless, we know from the ACE study and other epidemiologic research that violence—in all its forms—may represent the most common adversity and one of the biggest risk factors that children experience. As Donnelly and Goyal describe in this special issue, exposure to violence is common and often predisposes children to other adversities in the future.[17] This includes intimate partner violence, adolescent relationship abuse, community violence, gun violence (including suicide and mass shootings), bullying/cyber bullying, child maltreatment (ie, abuse and neglect), and media violence.[17] Furthermore, this burden is disproportionately borne by children with family histories of discriminatory redlining practices and environmental health disparities (lead poisoning), as well as ongoing exposure to overpolicing and systemic racism in our justice system, gentrification and housing inequalities, disparities in schools and afterschool activities, as well as neighborhood safety.

Something clearly must be done but addressing trauma due to violence without a methodical medical approach that is both evolution-informed and physiology-informed may not only be ineffective but also potentially harm inducing. TIC is the way to thread that needle. Asking about and responding to adversity experienced by patients requires adherence and a commitment to a TIC approach.[18]

IN CLINICAL PRACTICE
Violence and the Pathophysiology of Toxic Stress

Overall, the toll of violence on children in America is profound. TIC nudges pediatricians toward keeping toxic stress at the top of their minds. As noted earlier, toxic stress is the result of strong, frequent, or prolonged activation of our stress response system in the absence of buffering SSNRs.[19] Development of toxic stress is not dependent on the source or type of stress, rather, it depends on the magnitude and duration of each individual's biological response to the stressor. This is why the same stressor can influence people in different ways. It is particularly harmful for children when these biological disruptions persist during sensitive periods of development in the brain as well as in other organ systems because they can result in enduring structural changes and pathophysiology. We see impacts on areas of the brain including the prefrontal cortex, hippocampus, and amygdala and alterations in the immune response leading to inflammation and somatic effects. Ultimately, for children, this can lead to problems in learning, behavior, and both physical and mental health.

The nature of a child's stress response to an adverse event, including the meaning they make of that event,[4] is influenced by the interactive effects of the immediate exposures, earlier personal experiences, individual genetic predispositions, and developmental timing.[20] In this way, a complex constellation of genes, environment, and time embed adverse childhood experiences into developing children's biology. Pediatricians are uniquely positioned to address childhood trauma because of their ability to leverage their broad expertise in epidemiology, developmental psychology, neuroscience, and epigenetics.[21]

Trauma-Informed Care: Building the Buffering, Not Just Summing the Suffering

The goals of TIC are to, "assess, recognize and respond to the effects of traumatic experiences on children, caregivers and healthcare providers."[22] True TIC is about relationships and is rooted in the affiliate stress response. It is about applying empathy and engagement, connecting, and collaborating, and meeting the reality of our patients' lives. As described above, humans address stress and consequent morbidities best by turning toward each other and tending and befriending. Research bears this out repeatedly over time. Thus, *instead of just summing the suffering, pediatric trauma-informed care builds the buffering of relational health.*

Building the Buffering: Physiologic Foundations of Relational Health

Developmental science is only beginning to explain the way relational health buffers adversity and builds resilience but emerging data suggest that responsive interactions between children and engaged, attuned adults are paramount.[5,23–28] And this bears out beyond infancy into adulthood and even intergenerationally. For example, Peter Bos describes a neuroendocrine model that accounts for the intergenerational transmission of caregiving practices.[29] Other research describes how biobehavioral synchrony between parents and infants primes the brain and body to face the environment into which a child is born.[30]

Fundamentally, violence is a disruption of the SSNRs critical to child health. Being physically abused by a person we trust (eg, a significant other), or watching someone we are hardwired to care for get assaulted or injured (eg, parental intimate partner violence), or losing a loved one or best friend to gun violence are all examples of how violence disrupts or severs relationships. This largely explains the well-established associations between violence exposure and poor health outcomes decades later, and underscores the importance of understanding the biological mechanisms that allow adversity in childhood to "get under the skin" and negatively influence life-course trajectories.[23,31,32]

The good news is that just as adversity becomes embedded, so too can positive experiences lead to improved outcomes later in life.[25,26] For example, positive relational experiences, such as engaged, responsive caregivers,[33,34] or shared children's book reading,[35] are associated with positive impacts on learning, behavior, and health. Holding hands with a friend or loved one—as compared with a stranger—decreases the subjective feeling of pain in the form of electric shock.[36] Moreover, the Principal Investigators of the Harvard Study of Adult Development, which is the longest-running scientific study in human history (beginning in 1938), boil their research findings down to a single principle for living: "Good relationships keep us healthier and happier."[37] Not only do SSNRs buffer adversity and turn potentially toxic stress responses into tolerable or positive responses but they are also the primary vehicle for building the foundational resilience skills that allow children to cope with future adversity in an adaptive, healthy manner.[3,24] As such, relational health refers to the ability to form and maintain SSNR.[38–40]

These findings highlight the need for multigenerational (eg, "two-generation") approaches that support parents and adults as they, in turn, provide the SSNRs that all children need to flourish. The pediatrician can scaffold the development of SSNRs throughout all ages and developmental stages, including prenatally and postnatally, and from a baby's earliest days.[1,27,41,42] This can be done, for example, using universal primary preventions (such as positive parenting programs, Reach Out and Read Programs,[43,44] and developmentally appropriate play)[45] as well as more precise screening for relational health barriers such as maternal depression, food insecurity, or exposure to racism, as well as indicated treatments to address symptoms and repair strained or compromised relationships using evidence-based therapies (discussed more below).

Relational Health Builds Resilience

Pediatricians who "Build the Buffering" take a strengths-based approach by helping the patient identify and exercise their own resilience skills, which can be remembered using the THREADS acronym (**Table 1**). Resilience is defined as a dynamic process of positive adaptation to significant adversities.[22] This is not a static or innate individual quality but includes skills children learn over time with reliable support from dyadic attachment figures.

The development of resilience includes aptitudes that are attained through play, exploration, and exposure to a variety of normal activities and resources. Studies have shown that development can be robust, even in the face of severe adversity, if certain basic adaptational mechanisms of human development (resilience factors)

Table 1	
Adaptational mechanisms of resilience	
T	*Thinking*, learning, and problem-solving skills with opportunity for cognitive development
H	*Hope*, optimism, faith, belief in a future for oneself
R	*Regulation* (self-regulation, self-control of emotions, behaviors, attention, and impulses)
E	*Efficacy* perceived by self or society; has sense of coherence (life is comprehensible, manageable, and meaningful)
A	*Attachment* to a positive, competent adult (ie, SSNR)
D	*Development* of age-salient developmental tasks, *DNA* (heritable, polygenic sensitivity to context)
S	*Social* ecology, including people, places, and policies in which one lives and learns

Abbreviation: SSNR, safe, stable, nurturing relationship.

Data from Masten AS. Ordinary magic. Resilience processes in development. *Am Psychol.* 2001;56(3)227–238; Masten, A., Best, K., & Garmezy, N. (1990). Resilience and development: Contributions from the study of children who overcome adversity. Development and Psychopathology, 2(4), 425–444; Forkey H, Griffin J, Szilagyi M. *Childhood Trauma and Resilience: A Practical Guide.* Itasca, IL: American Academy of Pediatrics; 2021.

are protected and in good working order. These mechanisms include attachment to a safe, stable, and nurturing caregiver, cognitive development with opportunity for continued growth, mastery of age-salient developmental tasks, self-control or self-regulation, belief that life has meaning, hope for the future, a sense of self-efficacy, and a network of supportive relationships.[42] However, if those basic adaptational mechanisms or protective factors are absent or impaired before, during, or after the adversity, then the outcomes for children tend to be worse.[42]

DISCUSSION
Case Presentation

Jake is a 17-year-old male patient who arrived alone to clinic with 2 months of daily emesis, oftentimes in the morning before school. He feels weak after vomiting. The feeling of needing to vomit lingers for the rest of the day. Before this, he has otherwise been healthy. Upon entering the room, Jake appears healthy and typically developed.

Engagement

Creating an environment where the patient trusts the pediatrician and feels safe and seen is called, "Engagement." Engagement begins the moment our patients and their caregivers come through the door. Feeling safe and seen unlocks the patient's affiliative "tend and befriend" pathway. Particularly when the pediatrician suspects exposure to traumatic violence, *the first intervention is safety and helping the patient feel understood, or "seen."* Without it, obtaining the necessary history is not possible. This largely explains why the therapeutic relationship contributes as much, and sometimes more, to patient outcomes than the particular treatment method.[46,47]

One brief and actionable way to promote safety adapted from Baylin and Hughes, is the PACE acronym (**Table 2**).[48,49] Of note, safety is a fluid neurobiological process. If at any point in the visit, the patient does not feel safe or emotionally regulated, the pediatrician should return to the intervention of engagement.

Table 2	
Pediatricians can Engage Patients and Promote Feelings of Safety with PACE.	
Playfulness	Gentle tone, uses humor, has a relaxed demeanor
Acceptance	Maintain a nonjudgmental, no-shame, no-blame approach; Respect patient and caregiver thoughts and feelings
Curiosity	"I'm wondering about…"; "Tell me more about…". Follow child and/or caregiver cues by asking open-ended questions; attempt to understand the family's primary concerns or glean the meaning behind the behavior
Empathy	Help patients feel understood (seen and heard). Validate wide range of feelings; highlight protective value that many intense emotions serve for caregivers and children

Adapted from Baylin J, Hughes D. The Neurobiology of Attachment-Focused Therapy: Enhancing Connection & Trust in the Treatment of Children & Adolescents (Norton Series on Interpersonal Neurobiology). 1st ed. W. Norton & Company; 2016; with permission.

When health-care systems are designed counter to our biology, biology always wins. The pediatrician may be strapped for time but the patient's nervous system does not care that we are running behind in our daily schedule. In fact, the appearance of rushing during the visit may counteract engagement. Ultimately, the visit will be significantly less productive if our health-care systems are at odds with our evolutionary biological need for safety and empathy. It is our belief that both patients and pediatricians intuitively know this, and the way our medical system is antithetically designed is a major driver of burnout and distrust in medicine.

Symptoms of Toxic Stress

If there was one take-home point to consider for children exposed to violence it might be: *If you hear about symptoms, think trauma; If you hear about trauma, think symptoms.*[22,50] We feel confident that elevating trauma in your differential diagnosis will pay dividends for several reasons: (1) the experience of adversity is common; (2) the symptoms of trauma overlap with the symptoms of other common pediatric conditions[51,52]; and (3) failure to do so might lead to an incorrect or incomplete diagnosis and treatment, enabling the effects of trauma to further embed.[53–55]

Table 3	
Most common symptoms of trauma exposure	
F	*Frets* (anxiety and worry) and *fears* (eg, triggered by people, places, or things)
R	*Regulation* difficulties (Often upset, afraid, or sad; hyperactive, impulsive, inattentive, or easily gets into arguments or physical fights), disorders of behaviors or emotions
A	*Attachment* challenges; trouble feeling happiness, love, or trust; insecure attachment relationships with caregivers; poor peer relationships; feels alone even when around other people
Y	*Yucky* (somatic complaints eg, headaches, stomach aches, vomiting/diarrhea, skin rashes, tachycardia); *yawning* (sleep problems including bad dreams), and *yelling* (aggression, impulsivity)
E	*Educational* concerns (concentrating or paying attention) often due to developmental delays (especially cognitive, social-emotional, and communication)
D	*Defeated* (hopeless, lacks meaning or purpose in life), *depressed*, or *dissociated* (separated from reality of moment, out-of-body feeling)

Adapted from Forkey H, Griffin J, Szilagyi M. Childhood Trauma and Resilience: A Practical Guide. Itasca, IL: American Academy of Pediatrics; 2021; with permission.

Symptoms commonly found in children experiencing toxic stress can be remembered using the FRAYED acronym and are found in **Table 3**. Pediatricians should be concerned that a child is experiencing toxic stress when the THREADS (see **Table 1**) of resilience are FRAYED (see **Table 3**). For children, the primary consequences are in development and behavior. Although adult consequences of the chronically overactive inflammatory response explain many of the ACE Study results of disease burden, we see some impacts on physical health even in childhood. Inflammatory disorders such as asthma or metabolic syndrome are more common, and children can suffer from inflammatory effects, which results in a "sick syndrome" or a feeling of unwellness. This may account for the common somatic complaints of children experiencing exposure to violence.[56]

Building a Differential Diagnosis

Exposure to violence (and other traumas) can result not just in isolated symptoms but also in symptom constellations, or diagnoses. Most people are familiar with *posttraumatic stress disorder* (PTSD), which is a psychiatric diagnosis that can only be made when specific criteria are met regarding the number, duration, and intensity of symptoms are met after a person has experienced, witnessed, or learned of a close family member experiencing an event involving actual or threatened death, serious injury, or sexual violation.[57] This diagnosis applies to some children exposed to violence but many develop symptoms that do not meet the full criterial for PTSD that still benefit from identification and attention.

The term *complex trauma* is defined by the National Child Traumatic Stress Network as encompassing both a child's exposure to multiple interpersonal traumatic events and the broad, pervasive, and predictable impact this exposure has on the individual child.[58] Complex trauma can disrupt a child's bonding with caregivers, development, and a child's sense of themselves.

Another term for the effects of complex trauma *is developmental trauma disorder* (DTD). This term refers to a proposed diagnosis based on evidence that children exposed to complex trauma are at risk for severe disruptions in their development in the domains of emotion, physical health, attention, cognition, learning, behavior, interpersonal relationships, and development of a clear sense of self.[55,59–61] DTD formally describes problems in self-regulation that occur because of trauma-related developmental impairments. DTD symptoms overlap or co-occur with several PTSD symptoms but DTD involves a wider range of types of dysregulation and is more strongly related to complex trauma than PTSD.[62] This diagnosis was not included in the most recent version of the psychiatric Diagnosis and Statistical Manual (DSM) but is used by some researchers and providers in the mental health and medical communities.[55,63]

Adding to the challenge, violence and maltreatment may result in symptoms that mimic commonly diagnosed medical conditions (eg, depression). However, these symptoms are in fact a "phenotype" of the child's adaptation to *ecological* factors (so-called, ecophenotypes). Ecophenotypes fit within the boundaries of conventional mental or behavioral diagnoses (eg, depression, ADHD) but their pathophysiology are likely distinct and have a different illness trajectory (eg, earlier age of onset, greater symptom severity, more comorbidity, and greater risk for suicide) and respond differently to common treatments.[51,64] As such, children are often diagnosed with comorbid conditions, such as ADHD, anxiety, depression, or developmental and learning issues. A more detailed description of diagnoses that are commonly confused with trauma or comorbid is covered in the AAP clinical report "Children Exposed to Maltreatment: Assessment and the Role of Psychotropic Medication."[52]

Diagnostic Approach

Returning to our case

The sudden onset of daily emesis and his body feeling depleted was a symptom that concerned the provider for a possible traumatic event (or multiple ongoing events that started 2 months ago). After ruling out infection, marijuana or other drug-associated emesis, or other gastrointestinal and neurologic illnesses or conditions, the physician asked, "Did anything scary or upsetting happen before these symptoms began?" He disclosed his step-father hit him and the family kicked him out of the home. The physician screened for depression and PTSD, and the patient endorsed symptoms of both. The patient began to cry when he read the screening question about dissociation, and admitted to feeling like he was out of body sometimes.

After we have engaged the patient and family and identified concerning trauma history or FRAYED symptoms, we use surveillance and screening to gather more information to guide next steps.

Surveillance

Surveillance is, "a flexible, continuous process whereby knowledgeable professionals perform skilled observations of children during the provision of healthcare." Most pediatricians are familiar with developmental surveillance[65] but surveillance is not limited to just developmental concerns and can be used effectively with trauma concerns. Surveillance includes open-ended questions that allow us to ask about a patient or family's experience or symptoms. As they do so, the pediatrician keeps several things in mind, including the patient's development, the relationship between child and caregiver, risks to that relationship, exposures to violence, as well as the child and caregiver strengths. Because more than deficits (eg, ACEs and social determinants of health), it is a child's resilience, peer relationships, and family functioning that seem to be the most critical predictors of how an individual child will do.[25,33]

Questions can include the following:

- Has anything scary or upsetting happened since your last visit?[66]
- Has anyone come or gone from the household lately?[49,66]
- How were you raised and how do you want to raise your child?[49]

Screening

Screening tests are not diagnostic but they are used to assess risk factors for a targeted problem to identify children who may otherwise escape detection and benefit from more comprehensive evaluation and services. Ideally, a screening tool should be validated for the specific indication for which it is being used and, on the population, you are intending to use it with, it should also have a clear cutoff score. Because trauma *exposure* does not predict the development of symptoms in individual patients, we think screening for *symptoms* of toxic stress is the best approach we have currently to identify children experiencing toxic stress.

Several validated measures for trauma-specific symptoms have been developed. Some examples of trauma screening tools are below, which can be used when children have been exposed to violence. Of note, screening tools that include questions about thoughts of suicide are valuable because those who have experienced violence are more likely to consider and die from suicide than peers.[67–69]

1. The Pediatric Traumatic Stress Screening Tool[70]: A 15-question tool with decision support. The tool defines a potentially traumatic exposure and then asks 2 open-ended questions about recent or past exposures and 12 trauma symptom-specific questions followed by a suicide screen.

2. Child Trauma Screen[71]: The CTS is a brief, empirically derived trauma screening measure for children with strong predictive accuracy. A cut-point of 8 or greater on the CTS reactions score for parent report and a cut-point of 6 or greater for child report seem to be appropriate to maximize identification of youth likely experiencing clinical levels of PTSD symptoms who require comprehensive trauma-focused assessment to determine service need.

3. UCLA PTSD Reaction Index for DSM-5–Brief Form[72]: A short 11-item form identifying children at different levels of PTSD risk. Developed from a larger psychometrically sound clinician-administered assessment tool for PTSD in children and adolescents.

Treatment and Management of Toxic Stress

Returning to our case

After screening for suicidality and self-harm—which Jake denied—and seeing how many toxic stress-related symptoms he had after screening for depression and PTSD, the pediatrician normalized Jake's symptoms and engaged in relational care. They had Jake return to clinic the next week and gave Jake several relational and relaxation options, of which Jake was asked to choose two. Jake chose to (1) connect in small, informal ways with people he trusted and felt safe with and (2) to exercise at least twice per week. The pediatrician lightheartedly said, "I'm gonna hold you accountable–when I see you next week, I'm going to ask whether you did those two things." The next visit, Jake's emesis had decreased from 7 days a week to 3 times per week and his depression and PTSD screening scores—while still high—had improved.

Critically, the first step of management is to identify an emergency versus nonemergency situation. When dealing with trauma-like exposure to violence, its causes, or its consequences, consideration of whether a child may be emergently at risk requires assessment and response as a top priority. When it comes to violence in the home, such as physical abuse, referral to child protective services may be necessary and mandated. We acknowledge and take seriously the substantial concerns regarding bias in medicine in the reporting of children and families to protective services, in particular for families of color, leading to harm.[73] We share these major concerns and also must address the child's immediate safety needs.[74] Other immediate safety issues may arise when a consequence of trauma is self-harm or intent to injure others. Screening for suicidality, self-injury, or intent to harm others is included in TIC along with clear protocols for how to address positive endorsement of these issues.

After assessing safety, it is important to tell the patient that their bodies and brains have responded appropriately to situations involving danger and threat, and that their reactions are common and expected given their experiences. For many children and families affected by trauma, the message they receive is that they are damaged or, "bad kids," so validating them is often the first step in recovery. It is also worth mentioning to the patient, especially for children, that the brain is continually changing and growing, and can heal from these experiences. This initial step of normalizing and creating optimism or hope in the child's future brings them back to affiliate response from fight–flight–freeze. Moreover, the process of naming the concern and validating the experience is a powerful way to demonstrate the medical provider's commitment to the patient and builds trust.

After identifying that there are not immediate safety concerns and that the child's body has responded exactly the way it should have to trauma, pediatricians should assess which treatment approach would best serve their patient: primary, secondary, or tertiary prevention. Primary preventions are universally administered to all patients regardless of exposure to trauma and focus on how to universally promote the development and maintenance of SSNRs. Most pediatricians do this already, for example, through discussion of positive parenting techniques or promoting Reach out and Read.

Secondary prevention focuses on identifying patients at high risk for poor outcomes resulting from toxic stress responses, and potential individual, family, and community barriers to SSNRs. This can be addressed first by developing respectful and caring therapeutic relationships with patients, families.[23] The positive therapeutic relationship from the medical provider can reduce child and parent stress. Pediatric providers can offer caregivers (and older children) advice about 3 specific interventions to help a patient recover from trauma. The "3 R's" (reassuring, restoring routines, and regulating) are the first steps toward restoring resilience in a child exposed to violence demonstrating symptoms.

- *Reassuring:* Repeatedly reassuring a child or teen that they are safe and allowing the youth to express how they feel can restore a sense of safety. For preverbal or young children, the caregiver can offer additional physical contact with hugs, gentle touch, and rocking to reduce the stress response after a trauma. Children need to know they are safe and protected even when the caregiver is not present. Examples include having the child and caregiver share matched stuffed toys when separated at bedtime or during parent work hours, having the caregiver provide sticky notes with loving messages, offering the child a picture of the caregiver to keep in their pocket, or talking about how the caregiver and child are connected by an "invisible string" can all be used to remind the child of those reassuring connections.
- *Restoring Routines* is a practical step for caregivers to use after the chaos of a violent event. Unpredictability is extremely costly for children's energy-balance and is a driver of toxic stress. Guiding the caregiver to use verbal prompts and pictorial charts as visual cues of routines and encouraging well-defined mealtimes, sleep times, and standard rituals for bathing and bedtime can restore a sense of order.
- *Regulating* is a larger task and involves helping the child step down the fight or flight stress response. Over time, they become more practiced and efficient. Reassuring and routines start this process but anticipatory guidance can be offered in the office setting to enhance regulation:
  - Sharing relaxation techniques with caregivers and youth such as belly breathing, guided imagery, meditation, yoga, stretching, and massage can be helpful in reducing stress responses and symptoms. Advising about adequate sleep and exercise is also important.
  - Caregivers may be surprised by strong tantrums or unexpected reactions to seemingly innocuous events. Young children who have experienced violence often do not have the vocabulary or understanding of their own emotional states. Naming emotions, being emotional containers for children, and identifying triggers with children are ways caregivers can help them cope.
  - The pediatric provider can also make referrals to community resources for mindfulness programs, parenting support, and specific caregiver skill training that includes psychoeducation, cognitive coping, relaxation techniques, positive parenting strategies, and reframing. The pediatric provider can have a referral list for community providers, arrange the referral, or provide care coordination to facilitate family engagement with community resources. Regulation can take longer but often relates to children having tools to express how they feel.

Table 4
Common evidence-based attunement and trauma therapy/treatments and evidence-informed practices (organized by age)

Treatment or Practice	Abbreviation	Age Range, y	Modality
Child–parent psychotherapy	CPP	0–5	Parent–child dyad
Attachment and biobehavioral catch-up	ABC	6–48 mo	Individual caregiver and dyadic sessions
Parent child interaction therapy	PCIT	2–7	Parent–child dyad
Attachment, regulation, and competency framework	ARC	2–young adult	Individual, caregiver–child sessions
Trauma-focused cognitive behavioral therapy	TF-CBT	3–18	Individual, parent–child sessions; group therapy format available
Eye movement desensitization and reprocessing	EMDR	4 and up	Individual
Child and family traumatic stress intervention	CFTSI	7–18	Individual and caregiver sessions
Trauma affect regulation: guide for education and therapy for adolescents	TARGET-A	10–18	Individual sessions
Cognitive behavioral intervention for trauma in schools	CBITS	10–18 (5th-12th grade)	Group therapy (school-based)
Structured psychotherapy for adolescents responding to chronic stress	SPARCS	12–21	Group therapy (residential)

More information related to trauma-focused evidence-based therapy/treatment is available at the following websites: National Child Traumatic Stress Network (www.nctsn.org), Evidence-Based Practice Resource Center (www.samhsa.gov/ebp-resource-center).
Adapted from Forkey H, Griffin J, Szilagyi M. Childhood Trauma and Resilience: A Practical Guide. Itasca, IL: American Academy of Pediatrics; 2021. Page 162; with permission.

Tertiary prevention focuses on the evidence-based practices that treat toxic stress-related morbidities. Many children exposed to violence do not need evidence-based treatment (EBT) for trauma and will recover with the supports noted above. Indications for referral include a history of exposure to a violent or traumatic event and (1) the presence of trauma-related symptoms or (2) a marked change in functioning. In these circumstances, referral to evidence-based trauma, attachment, or parental attunement therapy practices is indicated.

Working with a mental health provider can help tease apart symptoms and afford the opportunity to best meet the needs of the child. Although full discussion of EBT is beyond the scope of this article, a simple table outlining various EBTs can be found below (**Table 4**).[49] Additionally see Kemal and colleague's article, "Mental Health and Violence," in this issue.[75] Additional resources can be found from the National Child Traumatic Stress Network and the Harvard Center for the Developing Child.

Burnout, Secondary Traumatic Stress, and Trauma-Informed Systems of Care

TIC recognizes that the health-care provider has their own stress response, especially when caring for children and families affected by violence. Finding opportunities to promote affiliate supports in the medical setting with colleagues and supervisors minimizes the potential for medical care to become traumatic or trigger trauma reactions in the provider, addresses distress, encourages positive coping, and provides anticipatory guidance regarding the recovery when exposure to trauma has affected the medical provider. When used in conjunction with family-centered practices, trauma-informed approaches enhance the quality of care for patients and their families and the well-being of medical professionals and support staff.[76,77]

SUMMARY

In the context of exposure to violence, preventing childhood toxic stress responses, promoting resilience, and optimizing development will require that all children be afforded the SSNRs that buffer these experiences and support development of foundational skills needed to cope with future adversity in an adaptive, health-promoting manner. Pediatricians may not recognize that they already use most of the principles of TIC.

When we meet a patient, we start with building a therapeutic relationship (engagement), we build a differential, and collaboratively create a treatment plan. In many ways, relational health and trauma should be treated similarly. Considering patient health and development in the context of the crucial role of the affiliate stress response and SSNRs allows the clinician to consider ways to promote health, and conversely the profound consequences of exposure to violence and other traumas. Epidemiologically, we know a pediatrician should presume that most of their patients experience trauma in some capacity.

When diagnosed, the best treatment we have for toxic stress is relational health, connecting our patients and their families to safe, stable, and nurturing people and organizations. Our aims should be to build a web of support—of which we pediatricians and our clinical staff are a thread—as an immediate brief intervention and, in the long run, hope to scaffold the child and their caregivers with emotional support and skills that ultimately help them buffer against this and other future traumas.

On top of this critical foundation, we layer secondary and tertiary level interventions as necessary, such as office-based suggestions (3R's), and referral to EBTs. Even then, a patient's willingness to engage in therapy often depends on their relationship and trust in the pediatrician recommending them. TIC starts and ends with the relationship.

CLINICS CARE POINTS

- TIC is fundamentally relational health care: Scaffolding the patient's ability to form and maintain SSNRs that allow the child to use the affiliate response to threat, including violence.
- The rapid brain development of the first years of life and the influence of attachment to a committed attuned caregiver provide both an explanation for a child's vulnerability to violence and an opportunity for resilience.
- Trauma symptoms can vary, from changes in eating and sleeping to more significant physical and mental health effects requiring mental health referral. Individual differences in trauma symptoms are largely due to variability in exposure and buffering of SSNRs as well as genetic variations influenced by the early environment.
- TIC is achieved using tools pediatricians already implement daily in their practice, starting with building trust (engagement), and providing a patient-centered and family-centered medical home where patients feel safe and seen.
- Diagnosis can often only be made if the pediatrician recognizes the variety of symptoms that result from exposure to violence and/or asks whether a patient has any of these symptoms when a patient discloses exposure to violence or other traumatic events.
- Treatment can begin in the office setting with psychoeducation and brief guidance for caregivers by, for example, using the 3 R's (reassure, return to routine, and regulation).
- Some children and families will benefit from warm handoffs to evidence-based trauma therapy or other community services to address symptoms and help restore or repair the relationships that may have been negatively influenced by the effects of violence.
- Wellness of the care team is of paramount importance if they are to help our patients and their families with this challenging work. Investing in safety and supportive relationships, decreasing stress, and promoting resilience for health-care personnel pays dividends.

DISCLOSURE

Supported in part by the National Center for Advancing TranslationalSciences of the National Institutes of Health under Award Numbers UL1TR002378 and TL1TR002382.

REFERENCES

1. Harvard Center for Developing Child. Three Early Childhood Development Principles to Improve Child Outcomes. https://developingchild.harvard.edu/resources/three-early-childhood-development-principles-improve-child-family-outcomes/. Accessed March 6, 2023.
2. Taylor SE. Tend and Befriend: Biobehavioral Bases of Affiliation Under Stress. Curr Dir Psychol Sci 2006;15(6):273–7.
3. Garner AS. Thinking Developmentally: Nurturing Wellness in Childhood to Promote Lifelong Health. https://doi.org/10.1542/9781610021531.
4. Tronick E, Beeghly M. Infants' meaning-making and the development of mental health problems. Am Psychol 2011;66(2):107–19.
5. Shonkoff JP, Garner AS. Committee on Psychosocial Aspects of Child and Family Health, Committee on Early Childhood, Adoption and DC, Section on Developmental and Behavioral Pediatrics. The lifelong effects of early childhood adversity and toxic stress. Pediatrics 2012;129(1):e232–46.
6. McEwen BS, Gianaros PJ. Central role of the brain in stress and adaptation: links to socioeconomic status, health, and disease. Ann N Y Acad Sci 2010;1186: 190–222.

7. Anda RF, Felitti VJ, Bremner JD, et al. The enduring effects of abuse and related adverse experiences in childhood. Eur Arch Psychiatry Clin Neurosci 2006; 256(3):174–86.

8. Merrick MT, Ford DC, Ports KA, et al. Vital Signs: Estimated Proportion of Adult Health Problems Attributable to Adverse Childhood Experiences and Implications for Prevention — 25 States, 2015–2017. MMWR Morb Mortal Wkly Rep 2019;68(44):999–1005.

9. Anda RF, Porter LE, Brown DW. Inside the Adverse Childhood Experience Score: Strengths, Limitations, and Misapplications. Am J Prev Med 2020; 59(2):293–5.

10. Siegel BS, Dobbins MI, Earls MF, et al. Early childhood adversity, toxic stress, and the role of the pediatrician: Translating developmental science into lifelong health. Pediatrics 2012;129(1). https://doi.org/10.1542/peds.2011-2662.

11. PACES Connection. Available at: https://www.pacesconnection.com/. Accessed January 27, 2023.

12. Bhushan D, Kotz K, McCall J, et al. Roadmap for Resilience: The California Surgeon General's Report on Adverse Childhood Experiences, Toxic Stress, and Health. Office of the California Surgeon General; 2020. https://doi.org/10.48019/PEAM8812.

13. Sherin KM, Stillerman AJ, Chandrasekar L, et al. Recommendations for Population-Based Applications of the Adverse Childhood Experiences Study: Position Statement by the American College of Preventive Medicine. AJPM Focus 2022;1(2):100039.

14. Campbell TL. Screening for adverse childhood experiences (ACEs) in primary care: a cautionary note. JAMA 2020;323(23):2379–80.

15. Finkelhor D. Screening for adverse childhood experiences (ACEs): Cautions and suggestions. Child Abuse Negl 2018;85:174–9.

16. Meehan AJ, Baldwin JR, Lewis SJ, et al. Poor Individual Risk Classification From Adverse Childhood Experiences Screening. Am J Prev Med 2022;62(3):427–32.

17. Goyal M, Donnelly K. Epidemiology of violence experienced by children. Pediatr Clin North Am 2023. Addressing violence in pediatric practice.

18. Racine N, Killam T, Madigan S. Trauma-Informed Care as a Universal Precaution: Beyond the Adverse Childhood Experiences Questionnaire. JAMA Pediatr 2020; 174(1):5–6.

19. DeVoe JE, Geller A, Negussie Y, editors. Vibrant and healthy kids. Washington, D.C.: National Academies Press; 2019.

20. Boyce WT, Levitt P, Martinez FD, et al. Genes, Environments, and Time: The Biology of Adversity and Resilience. Pediatrics 2021;147(2). https://doi.org/10.1542/peds.2020-1651.

21. Shonkoff JP, Garner AS, Siegel BS, et al. The lifelong effects of early childhood adversity and toxic stress. Pediatrics 2012;129(1). https://doi.org/10.1542/peds.2011-2663.

22. Forkey H, Szilagyi M, Kelly ET, et al. Trauma-Informed Care. Pediatrics 2021; 148(2). e2021052580.

23. Garner A, Yogman M, Committee on psychosocial aspects of child and family health, section on developmental and behavioral pediatrics COEC. Preventing Childhood Toxic Stress: Partnering With Families and Communities to Promote Relational Health. Pediatrics 2021;148(2). https://doi.org/10.1542/peds.2021-052582.

24. National Scientific Council on the Developing Child. Supportive relationships and active skill-building strengthen the foundations of resilience: working paper No.

13. Cambridge, MA: National Scientific Council on the Developing Child; 2015. Available at: https://developingchild.harvard.edu/resources/supportive-relationships-and-active-skill-building-strengthen-the-foundations-of-resilience/. Accessed March 14, 2023.

25. Bethell C, Jones J, Gombojav N, et al. Positive Childhood Experiences and Adult Mental and Relational Health in a Statewide Sample: Associations Across Adverse Childhood Experiences Levels. JAMA Pediatr 2019;173(11):e193007.

26. Sege RD, Harper Browne C. Responding to ACEs With HOPE: Health Outcomes From Positive Experiences. Acad Pediatr 2017;17(7S):S79–85.

27. Garner AS, Forkey H, Szilagyi M. Translating Developmental Science to Address Childhood Adversity. Acad Pediatr 2015;15(5):493–502.

28. Feldman R. The Neurobiology of Human Attachments. Trends Cogn Sci 2017; 21(2):80–99.

29. Bos PA. The endocrinology of human caregiving and its intergenerational transmission. Dev Psychopathol 2017;29(3):971–99.

30. Feldman R. Sensitive periods in human social development: New insights from research on oxytocin, synchrony, and high-risk parenting. Dev Psychopathol 2015;27(2):369–95.

31. Hertzman C. Putting the concept of biological embedding in historical perspective. Proc Natl Acad Sci U S A 2012;109(Suppl 2):17160–7.

32. McEwen BS. Brain on stress: how the social environment gets under the skin. Proc Natl Acad Sci U S A 2012;109(Suppl 2):17180–5.

33. Bethell CD, Gombojav N, Whitaker RC. Family Resilience And Connection Promote Flourishing Among US Children. Even Amid Adversity. Health Aff (Millwood) 2019;38(5):729–37.

34. Hambrick EP, Brawner TW, Perry BD, et al. Beyond the ACE score: Examining relationships between timing of developmental adversity, relational health and developmental outcomes in children. Arch Psychiatr Nurs 2019;33(3):238–47.

35. Mendelsohn AL, Cates CB, Weisleder A, et al. Reading Aloud, Play, and Social-Emotional Development. Pediatrics 2018;141(5). https://doi.org/10.1542/peds.2017-3393.

36. Coan JA, Beckes L, Gonzalez MZ, et al. Relationship status and perceived support in the social regulation of neural responses to threat. Soc Cogn Affect Neurosci 2017;12(10):1574–83.

37. Waldinger R, Schulz M. The good life: lessons from the world's longest scientific study of happiness. Simon & Schuster; 2023. p. 352.

38. A FrameWorks Strategic Brief in collaboration with the Center for the Study of Social Policy. Building Relationships: Framing Early Relational Health.

39. Slopen N, McLaughlin KA, Shonkoff JP. Interventions to improve cortisol regulation in children: a systematic review. Pediatrics 2014;133(2):312–26.

40. Jaffee SR, Bowes L, Ouellet-Morin I, et al. Safe, stable, nurturing relationships break the intergenerational cycle of abuse: a prospective nationally representative cohort of children in the United Kingdom. J Adolesc Health 2013;53(4 Suppl):S4–10.

41. Traub F, Boynton-Jarrett R. Modifiable Resilience Factors to Childhood Adversity for Clinical Pediatric Practice. Pediatrics 2017;139(5). https://doi.org/10.1542/peds.2016-2569.

42. Forkey H, Szilagyi M, Kelly ET, et al. Trauma-Informed Care. Pediatrics 2021; 148(2). https://doi.org/10.1542/peds.2021-052580.

43. Zuckerman B. Promoting early literacy in pediatric practice: twenty years of reach out and read. Pediatrics 2009;124(6):1660–5.

44. Zuckerman B, Needlman R. 30 Years of Reach Out and Read: Need for a Developmental Perspective. Pediatrics 2020;145(6). https://doi.org/10.1542/peds.2019-1958.

45. Weisleder A, Cates CB, Dreyer BP, et al. Promotion of Positive Parenting and Prevention of Socioemotional Disparities. Pediatrics 2016;137(2):e20153239.

46. Norcross JC, Lambert MJ. Relationship science and practice in psychotherapy: closing commentary. Psychotherapy 2014;51(3):398–403.

47. Finset A, Ørnes K. Empathy in the Clinician-Patient Relationship: The Role of Reciprocal Adjustments and Processes of Synchrony. J patient Exp 2017; 4(2):64–8.

48. Baylin J, Hughes D. The Neurobiology of attachment-focused therapy: enhancing connection & trust in the treatment of children & adolescents (Norton Series on interpersonal neurobiology). 1st edition. W. Norton & Company; 2016.

49. Forkey H, Griffin J, Szilagyi M. Childhood trauma and resilience: a practical guide. American Academy of Pediatrics; 2021.

50. Forkey H. Putting Your Trauma Lens On. Pediatr Ann 2019;48(7):e269–73.

51. Teicher MH, Samson JA. Childhood maltreatment and psychopathology: A case for ecophenotypic variants as clinically and neurobiologically distinct subtypes. Am J Psychiatry 2013;170(10):1114–33.

52. Keeshin B, Forkey HC, Fouras G, et al. American academy of pediatrics, council on child abuse and neglect, council on foster care, adoption, and kinship care, american academy of child and adolescent psychiatry, committee on child maltreatment and violence COAAFC. Children Exposed to Maltreatment: Assessment and the Role of Psychotropic Medication. Pediatrics 2020;145(2). https://doi.org/10.1542/peds.2019-3751.

53. Stein REK, Storfer-Isser A, Kerker BD, et al. Beyond ADHD: How Well Are We Doing? Acad Pediatr 2016;16(2):115–21.

54. Heneghan A, Stein REK, Hurlburt MS, et al. Mental health problems in teens investigated by U.S. child welfare agencies. J Adolesc Health 2013;52(5):634–40.

55. Ford JD, Grasso D, Greene C, et al. Clinical significance of a proposed developmental trauma disorder diagnosis: results of an international survey of clinicians. J Clin Psychiatry 2013;74(8):841–9.

56. Danese A, Moffitt TE, Harrington H, et al. Adverse childhood experiences and adult risk factors for age-related disease: depression, inflammation, and clustering of metabolic risk markers. Arch Pediatr Adolesc Med 2009;163(12):1135–43.

57. American Psychiatric Association. Diagnostic and Statistical manual of mental disorders. 5th edition. American Psychiatric Association; 2013.

58. Complex Trauma | The National Child Traumatic Stress Network. Available at: https://www.nctsn.org/what-is-child-trauma/trauma-types/complex-trauma. Accessed March 28, 2023.

59. Bremness A, Polzin W. Commentary: Developmental Trauma Disorder: A Missed Opportunity in DSM V. J Can Acad Child Adolesc Psychiatry 2014;23(2):142–5. http://www.ncbi.nlm.nih.gov/pubmed/24872830.

60. Sar V. Developmental trauma, complex PTSD, and the current proposal of DSM-5. Eur J Psychotraumatol 2011;2. https://doi.org/10.3402/ejpt.v2i0.5622.

61. Spinazzola J, van der Kolk B, Ford JD. Developmental Trauma Disorder: A Legacy of Attachment Trauma in Victimized Children. J Trauma Stress 2021;34(4): 711–20.

62. Schmid M, Petermann F, Fegert JM. Developmental trauma disorder: pros and cons of including formal criteria in the psychiatric diagnostic systems. BMC Psychiatr 2013;13:3.

63. Anda RF, Felitti VJ, Bremner JD, et al. The enduring effects of abuse and related adverse experiences in childhood. A convergence of evidence from neurobiology and epidemiology. Eur Arch Psychiatry Clin Neurosci 2006;256(3):174–86.

64. MH T, SL A, A P, et al. The neurobiological consequences of early stress and childhood maltreatment. Neurosci Biobehav Rev 2003;27(1–2):33–44.

65. Garg A, Dworkin PH. Applying surveillance and screening to family psychosocial issues: implications for the medical home. J Dev Behav Pediatr 2011;32(5): 418–26.

66. Cohen JA, Kelleher KJ, Mannarino AP. Identifying, treating, and referring traumatized children: the role of pediatric providers. Arch Pediatr Adolesc Med 2008; 162(5):447–52.

67. Thompson MP, Kingree JB, Lamis D. Associations of adverse childhood experiences and suicidal behaviors in adulthood in a U.S. nationally representative sample. Child Care Health Dev 2019;45(1):121–8.

68. Poindexter EK, Mitchell SM, Brown SL, et al. Interpersonal Trauma and Suicide Ideation: The Indirect Effects of Depressive Symptoms, Thwarted Belongingness, and Perceived Burden. J Interpers Violence 2022;37(1–2):NP551–70.

69. Yoo Y, Park H-J, Park S, et al. Interpersonal trauma moderates the relationship between personality factors and suicidality of individuals with posttraumatic stress disorder. PLoS One 2018;13(1):e0191198.

70. Keeshin B, Byrne K, Thorn B, et al. Screening for Trauma in Pediatric Primary Care. Curr Psychiatry Rep 2020;22(11):60.

71. Lang JM, Connell CM. Development and validation of a brief trauma screening measure for children: The Child Trauma Screen. Psychol Trauma 2017;9(3):390–8.

72. Rolon-Arroyo B, Oosterhoff B, Layne CM, et al. The UCLA PTSD Reaction Index for DSM-5 Brief Form: A Screening Tool for Trauma-Exposed Youths. J Am Acad Child Adolesc Psychiatry 2020;59(3):434–43.

73. Morgan W, Schultz KV, Adiba A, et al. Promoting Resiliency and Eliminating Disparities-Best Practices when Working with Child Welfare Involved Youth of Color. Child Adolesc Psychiatr Clin N Am 2022;31(4):631–48.

74. Forkey HC, Morgan W, Schwartz K, et al. Outpatient Clinic Identification of Trauma Symptoms in Children in Foster Care. J Child Fam Stud 2016;25(5):1480–7.

75. Kemal S, Nwabuo A, Hoffmann J. Mental health and violence. Pediatr Clin North Am 2023. Addressing Violence in Pediatric PracNce.

76. Marsac ML, Kassam-Adams N, Hildenbrand AK, et al. Implementing a Trauma-Informed Approach in Pediatric Health Care Networks. JAMA Pediatr 2016; 170(1):70–7.

77. Stubbe DE. Optimizing Empathy: Physician Self-Care as a Crucial Component of Trauma-Informed Treatment. Focus 2017;15(4):432–4.

Mental Health and Violence in Children and Adolescents

Samaa Kemal, MD, MPH[a,b,*], Adaobi Nwabuo, MBBS, MPH[c],
Jennifer Hoffmann, MD, MS[a,b]

KEYWORDS

- Mental health • Violence • Pediatrics • Perpetration • Victimization

KEY POINTS

- Children with mental illness are at increased risk for violence victimization, and, although most children with mental illness are nonviolent, there are specific types of mental illness that may be associated with the development of violent behavior.
- Children exposed to violence have an increased risk of developing mental health symptoms thereafter regardless of whether violence exposure is direct (eg, assault, adolescent relationship aggression, or abuse) or indirect (eg, intimate partner violence or community violence).
- Pediatric clinicians can use validated screening tools to assess for violence exposure and mental health symptoms among children, and, for those children who screen positive, clinicians should provide referrals to trauma-informed, culturally competent, and evidence-based therapies.

The relationship between mental health and violence in children is complex. It is known that some children with mental health conditions may be at higher risk for violence victimization or violence perpetration. Alternatively, violence exposure and victimization may themselves precipitate adverse mental health outcomes.

Mental health conditions are common among US children. Approximately 1 in 6 children in the United States has a mental health disorder.[1,2] Suicide is the second leading cause of death among children ages 10 to 14 and the third leading cause of death for adolescents and young adults ages 15 to 24.[3] During the coronavirus disease 2019 (COVID-19) pandemic, leading pediatric professional organizations declared a national emergency in youth mental health.[4] During this time, firearm sales reached

[a] Division of Emergency Medicine, Ann & Robert H. Lurie Children's Hospital of Chicago, 225 East Chicago Avenue, Box 62, Chicago, IL 60611, USA; [b] Department of Pediatrics, Northwestern University Feinberg School of Medicine, 420 East Superior Street, Chicago, IL 60611, USA; [c] Department of Psychiatry and Behavioral Sciences, University of California Davis Health, 2230 Stockton Boulevard, Sacramento, CA 95817, USA
* Corresponding author. Emergency Department, Ann & Robert H. Lurie Children's Hospital of Chicago, 225 East Chicago Avenue, Box 62, Chicago, IL 60611.
E-mail address: skemal@luriechildrens.org

Pediatr Clin N Am 70 (2023) 1201–1215
https://doi.org/10.1016/j.pcl.2023.06.011
0031-3955/23/© 2023 Elsevier Inc. All rights reserved.

the highest level ever recorded in US history,[5] and firearm-related pediatric hospital encounters increased significantly.[6] The pandemic also brought with it a higher burden of family violence[7] and increased severity of child abuse-related injuries.[8] With rising rates of mental health disorders and violence in children, examination of the relationship between the two is timely.

Moreover, the authors acknowledge that similar upstream risk factors and environmental circumstances may increase the risk for violence involvement and the risk of adverse mental health outcomes[9] as seen in children who have experienced adverse childhood experiences (ACEs) and children from communities with a history of structural marginalization.[10] It is critically important for pediatric clinicians to recognize how various individual and community-level factors may place a child at risk for adverse mental health outcomes, in addition to violence victimization and/or perpetration. Thus, in this article, the authors aim to examine the complex interplay between mental health and violence in children.

MENTAL HEALTH AS A RISK FACTOR FOR VIOLENCE VICTIMIZATION AND PERPETRATION
Mental Health and Violence Victimization

Most people with mental illness are more likely to be victims of violence than perpetrators.[11,12] Adults with serious mental illness experience an 11-fold higher rate of violence victimization than the general population, even after adjusting for demographic differences.[13] Among children and adolescents, mental health problems also increase the risk of violence victimization. For example, 1 study conducted using a national probability sample of 1467 children ages 2 to 17 found that children with high levels of co-occurring internalizing and externalizing symptoms have increased exposure to several forms of violence victimization, including peer victimization, maltreatment, and sexual victimization. This increased risk of victimization persists after controlling for earlier victimization and adversity.[14] Among children with mental health symptoms, the type of victimization varies by age, with elementary school-age children experiencing more peer victimization and adolescents experiencing higher rates of sexual victimization.[14]

Mental Health and Violence Perpetration

Most people with mental illnesses are nonviolent. Although higher rates of violence perpetration have been identified among people with serious mental illness, the rate of violent behavior only increases from 2% for the general public to 5% for adults with serious mental illness.[15] In adjusted models, severe mental illness alone did not predict future violence, although co-occurring severe mental illness with substance use and past history of violence are independently associated with future violence.[16] Notably, only a small proportion of all violent acts are committed by people with mental illness. For instance, a study of violent incidents in the United States over a 1-year period found that only 3% of violent offenders had schizophrenia.[17] Similarly, an analysis of violent incidents in England and Wales from 2015 to 2016 estimated that 5.3% were committed by individuals with severe mental illness.[18] Clearly, most violent acts are carried out by people without mental illnesses.

Most children with mental health conditions are not violent, but some types of mental illness have been associated with some forms of aggressive behavior. Child oppositional defiant and antisocial behaviors have been associated with violence and aggression, but many studies on this relationship have been limited to specific high-risk populations (such as justice-involved youth) or do not adequately account for shared family and community factors.[19] In 1 study, half of justice-involved youth were found to have substance use disorders; over 40% met criteria for disruptive behavior disorders, and more than 20% of girls met criteria for a major depressive episode.[20] In a longitudinal community-based study in Chicago, oppositional defiant problems were the only mental health condition that significantly predicted future violence, after adjusting for individual-, peer-, family-, and neighborhood-level variables.[21] In considering these results, it is important to recognize that clinician and systemic biases contribute to the overdiagnosis of oppositional defiant disorder among children of color, whereas these behaviors may actually be related to trauma exposures or alternative mental health diagnoses.[22,23]

One approach to understanding the complex relationship between mental health conditions and violence involves studying sibling pairs, who share similar genetics and environments. In a large population-based sample of US youth, ACEs were significantly associated with childhood antisocial behavior, adolescent delinquency, and young adult violent victimization in bivariate analyses.[24] However, after using sibling comparisons to adjust for unmeasured common genetic and shared environmental confounders, siblings exposed to more ACEs did not demonstrate higher levels of antisocial behavior, delinquent behavior, or risk for future victimization. This suggests that shared familial and environmental factors may underpin child outcomes.

Autism spectrum disorder (ASD) can in some situations be associated with aggression; it is important to note that this aggression most often impacts within-family functioning and well-being.[25] In a sample of 1584 children and adolescents with ASD enrolled in the Autism Treatment Network, 53% were reported to have aggressive behaviors.[26] In inpatient medical units, episodes of acute agitation occur during as many as 12% of hospitalizations by children with ASD.[27] Specific therapeutic strategies such as functional behavioral assessment, reinforcement strategies, and functional communication training may reduce the frequency and intensity of aggressive behaviors among children with ASD.[28] Pharmacologic treatments, particularly second-generation antipsychotic agents, may also be of some benefit in reducing aggression among children with ASD.[28]

Assessment of Violence Risk and Prevention

To prevent violence perpetration among children with mental health disorders, tools are needed to identify risk. To this end, some tools have been developed to predict violence within health care settings and schools. Among children admitted to inpatient psychiatric units, the Brief Rating of Aggression by Children and Adolescents (BRACHA) accurately and reliably predicts the risk of violence during hospitalization.[29,30] It consists of 14 items (12 historical and behavioral items and 2 clinical observations) scored by emergency department staff before admission. Efforts have also been made to predict risks of school violence. For instance, an analysis of structured interviews with students using natural language processing and machine learning demonstrated capacity to predict risks of school violence.[31] Such risk assessment tools are not yet widely used.

Once a child has been identified as at risk for violence perpetration, effective preventive interventions are needed to mitigate risk. Improved access to mental health services is likely to be important, as half of children with mental health disorders in the United States do not receive needed treatment or counseling from mental health professionals.[2] Additionally, evidence-based violence prevention interventions have been developed for families, schools, and communities.[32] Examples include programs to enhance parent-child bonding and to promote community-based mentorship.[32]

Multiple interventions targeted to various developmental stages and levels (both individual- and population-based) may be needed to prevent violence.[33]

MENTAL HEALTH FOLLOWING EXPOSURE TO VIOLENCE

Adverse mental health outcomes following exposure to violence are common in youth.[34,35] It is important to consider the nuanced ways in which direct and indirect exposures to violence affect youth. Direct violence exposures are defined as personal experiences of violence victimization through threat or injury.[36] Examples of direct violence exposures in children include assault, adolescent relationship aggression, and child abuse. Indirect violence exposures are defined as witnessing violence, hearing violence (eg, gunshots heard in the neighborhood), or losing a family member or peer as a victim of violence.[36] Examples of indirect violence exposures in children include intimate partner violence and community violence. All violence exposures, whether direct or indirect, may lead to mental health sequelae in youth, although effects may differ based on the type of exposure.[36,37]

Firearm Violence

Firearm injuries are associated with short- and long-term mental health sequelae among youth.[34] In 1 retrospective cohort study, over a quarter of youth with a firearm injury were diagnosed with a new mental health condition in the year after injury.[38] Compared with youth who sustain other types of traumatic injuries (ie, motor vehicle collisions), youth with firearm injuries have 1.5 times higher odds of developing new mental health diagnoses in the year after injury.[39] The most common mental health disorders that arise among youth after firearm injuries are substance-related and addictive disorders and trauma- or stressor-related disorders.[38,40] In particular, firearm-related injuries are strongly correlated with subsequent development of post-traumatic stress disorder (PTSD) in youth.[34,41] Youth with nonfatal firearm injuries also experience significant increases in mental health service utilization and expenditures following injury.[42,43]

Childhood exposure to firearm violence has been associated with the development of externalizing symptoms,[44] such as aggressive and disruptive behaviors, as well as internalizing symptoms,[45,46] such as anxiety and depression. Studies have suggested that younger children exposed to firearm violence may exhibit more internalizing symptoms, whereas older children may exhibit more externalizing symptoms.[36] The effects of exposure to firearm violence may differ based on age and developmental stage. One study found that younger children (ages 2–9 years) developed PTSD symptoms from indirect exposures (eg, hearing gun shots), while older children (ages 10–17 years) did not develop significant PTSD symptoms unless they were direct victims of gun violence.[41]

Child Abuse

ACEs, including childhood physical, sexual, and emotional abuse, are strongly correlated with adverse mental health outcomes during childhood and into adulthood. One systematic review and meta-analysis found that adults who experienced multiple ACEs were more likely to have depression, anxiety, suicide attempts, problematic alcohol use, and problematic drug use.[10] The cumulative effect of maltreatment among children has also been demonstrated, with increased mental health symptom severity as children experience more types of maltreatment.[47] Children who experience abuse have a high prevalence of PTSD, with reported incidence rates of up to 50% to 90%.[48] These children are also more likely to exhibit both internalizing and externalizing symptoms.[48,49] For example, a meta-analysis found that sexual and physical abuse are strongly associated with development of major depressive disorder (MDD) before age 18.[35] Experiences with childhood maltreatment throughout the life course appear to have independent and additive effects on children's mental health.

Adolescent Relationship Aggression

Adolescent relationship aggression (ARA) is highly prevalent among adolescents, with rates of 9% to 20% reported in nationally representative samples, and it is associated with subsequent mental health risks.[50–52] In particular, both boys and girls who experience ARA have increased risk of suicide attempts, while girls are also 2 times as likely to have severe depressive symptoms following ARA.[50,52] One study found that girls with depression and a history of ARA victimization were 61% more likely to attempt suicide than nonvictimized girls with depression.[53] Additionally, adolescents who experience more distinct forms of ARA (eg, sexual, physical, or psychological) are more likely to have adverse mental health outcomes, including depressive symptoms, suicide attempts, and substance abuse.[54,55] Given the prevalence of ARA among adolescents, pediatric clinicians may consider screening for ARA exposure to increase recognition of at-risk youth.[56]

Intimate Partner Violence

The negative impact of intimate partner (domestic) violence (IPV) on youth mental health outcomes is well described. In a meta-analysis of psychosocial outcomes, 63% of children exposed to IPV had worse emotional health outcomes compared with nonexposed children.[57] Youth who witness severe IPV are almost 3 times more likely to develop conduct disorder,[58] twice as likely to develop MDD,[35] and over 4 times more likely to have symptoms of anxiety.[59] Exposure to domestic violence provides a key example of how indirect violence exposure can be associated with pediatric mental health outcomes.

Community Violence

The isolated influence of community violence exposure on youth mental health is difficult to measure, given significant overlap with other family and neighborhood characteristics.[36] Studies have demonstrated that closer geographic proximity to violent events is associated with increased mental health symptoms and greater mental health service utilization after an event.[60,61] Youth who are chronically exposed to community violence may become desensitized and develop externalizing behaviors.[62] Among Black, urban adolescents, community violence exposure has also been associated with subsequent suicidal thoughts and behaviors.[63] Notably, community violence, and, in particular, firearm violence, disproportionately impacts communities of color as a result of historic trauma, systemic racism, and selective disinvestment in these communities.[64] With acute and chronic sequelae, the mental health consequences of community violence among youth are longitudinal and multifaceted.

MENTAL HEALTH SERVICE UTILIZATION

Many children who are exposed to violence face barriers to accessing mental health services. One national study identified that 20% of adolescents have experienced personal victimization, yet only half of those adolescents accessed mental health services within a year of trauma.[65] Another nationally representative study showed that 16% of children have experienced high ACE scores (defined as 5 or more ACEs for ages 2–9

Table 1
Screening and diagnostic tools for post-traumatic stress disorder

Screening or Diagnostic Tool	Purpose	Symptom Domains	Completed By	Target Age	Number of Items	Average Time to Complete
Child Behavior Checklist (CBCL)[90]	Screening	Social functioning, anxiety, mood, externalizing symptoms	Parent/caretaker	6–18	120	15 min
Child Trauma Screen (CTS)[91]	Screening	Trauma exposure, traumatic stress	Self	6–17	10	10 min
UCLA PTSD Reaction Index (UCLA PTSD RI)[92]	Screening/preliminary diagnosis	Traumatic stress, neglect	Self	6–18	48	10 min
Child PTSD Symptoms Scale – Self-Report Version for DSM-5 (CPSS-5-SR)[93]	Diagnostic	PTSD, daily functioning	Self	8–18	24	10 min

Abbreviation: PTSD, Post-traumatic stress disorder.

Table 2
Selected examples of treatment approaches for children exposed to violence

Treatment Approach	Overview	Target Age	Trauma Sub-type	Goals/Outcomes	Evidence Rating[a]
Trauma-Focused Cognitive-Behavioral Therapy (TF-CBT)[89]	An evidence-based treatment for children and adolescents impacted by trauma and their parents or caregivers A components-based treatment model that incorporates trauma-sensitive interventions with cognitive-behavioral, family, and humanistic principles and techniques	3–21	Sexual abuse, domestic violence, traumatic grief, disaster, terrorism, multiple or complex traumas	• Reduction in depressive, anxiety, post-traumatic stress symptoms • Reduction in parental distress	1
Child Parent Psychotherapy (CPP)[94]	CPP is based in attachment theory whose goal is to support and strengthen the child-caregiver relationship to restore the child's cognitive, behavioral, and social functioning	0–6	Loss or separation, community violence, medical conditions	• Reduction in behavioral problems • Improvement in depressive and PTSD symptoms • Improving change in attachment classification	2
Collaborative Models[72]	A practice team of primary care and behavioral health clinicians work in concert to provide a systematic, cost-effective, and patient- and family-centered approach	0+	All types	• Improvement in clinical outcomes • Early identification of symptoms	NR

(continued on next page)

Table 2
(continued)

Treatment Approach	Overview	Target Age	Trauma Sub-type	Goals/Outcomes	Evidence Rating[a]
	Model types are: consultation (formal and informal); colocation; and collaborative/ integrative (comanagement of cases)				
Hospital-based Violence Intervention Programs (HVIPs)[70]	Aim to reduce violent injury recidivism by providing intensive case management services to high-risk patients who were violently injured Holistically address risk factors for violent injury including mental health	Varies by program	Penetrating trauma, sexual trauma	• Reduce repeat injury • Access to longitudinal mental health services • Reduction in post-traumatic stress symptoms	NR
Structured Psychotherapy for Adolescents Responding to Chronic Stress (SPARCS)[95]	Manually-guided and empirically supported group treatment, primarily based on cognitive-behavioral principles. Teaches skills to improve resilience	12–21	Complex trauma, chronic traumas, chronic medical conditions	• Remaining in treatment • Improvement in post-traumatic stress symptoms	NR

Abbreviation: PTSD, post-traumatic stress disorder.

[a] California Evidence-Based Clearinghouse (CEBC) rating[96]. 1. Well-supported by research evidence. 2. Supported by research evidence. 3. Promising research evidence. 4. Evidence fails to demonstrate effect. 5. Concerning practice. NR. not able to be rated.

and 7 or more ACEs for ages 10–17), yet fewer than 50% had accessed mental health services within the last year.[66] Discrepancies in parent-child report of traumatic exposures may be 1 factor impeding identification of needs and referral for services.[67–69] At times, violent injury can serve as the point of access to mental health services, as is the case with Hospital-Based Violence Intervention Programs (HVIPs),[70,71] collaborative models,[72] and school-based interventions.[73]

Inequities in Access to Mental Health Services

Significant differences exist by race and ethnicity in the utilization of mental health services, with lower utilization among non-Hispanic Black and Hispanic children compared with non-Hispanic White children.[74–76] Specifically among children who have experienced ACEs such as violence exposure, fewer Black children receive mental health services compared with White children.[66] Proposed mechanisms underlying these inequities include differences in insurance coverage,[77] institutional mistrust,[78] stigma,[79] cultural misalignment between providers and clients,[80] lack of awareness of available services,[81] and differences in physician referrals.[82]

Multilayered efforts are needed to improve equity in access to mental health services among children exposed to violence. At an individual level, clinicians should select therapies to address trauma symptoms that are aligned with each child's individual, social, and cultural needs.[83,84] At a structural level, critical steps will include addressing structural determinants of health such as poverty, eliminating discriminatory practices, and increasing insurance access.[85]

Screening for Trauma Exposure and Interventions

The role of primary care pediatric clinicians in identifying and addressing potentially traumatic events and PTSD symptoms cannot be overemphasized.[86] For trauma-exposed youth, relational health and resilience can be improved through delivery of trauma-informed care, defined by the National Child Traumatic Stress Network as medical care in which all parties assess, recognize, and respond to the effects of traumatic stress on children, caregivers, and health care providers.[87] The framework of healing-centered engagement expands on this with a holistic strengths-based approach to healing that is focused on sustaining well-being.[88] Using trauma-informed care with a healing-centered approach, pediatric clinicians can learn about their patient's trauma exposure, assess for sequelae, and refer to mental health services when indicated. Several validated questionnaires have been developed to guide efforts to assess the impact of trauma (**Table 1**). Alternatively, pediatric clinicians can simply ask, "Has anything scary or concerning happened to you or your child since the last visit?"[87] If screening suggests exposure to a potentially traumatic event or PTSD symptoms, a referral to trauma-focused cognitive-behavioral therapy[89] or other evidence-based therapies may be indicated (**Table 2**). Pediatric clinicians can also provide contained relaxation tools such as deep breathing, mindfulness exercises, and reassurance.[87]

SUMMARY

In summary, the relationships between mental health and violence in youth are complex. Although some mental health conditions are associated with violence perpetration, most children with mental illness are nonviolent. In contrast, mental health conditions are a strong risk factor for violence victimization. In turn, children with a history of violence victimization are at higher risk for having mental health sequelae. Although the type of exposure to violence and age of exposure may influence symptom development, many children will develop internalizing and/or externalizing symptoms following direct exposures to violence. Importantly, indirect exposures to violence, such as intimate partner violence and community violence, can also lead to adverse mental health outcomes in children. Despite high rates of exposure to violence and mental health conditions among children, evidence-based mental health treatments for trauma- and stressor-related conditions remain underutilized, with notable inequities among Black and Hispanic children. It is critical that pediatric clinicians regularly screen youth for exposure to and risk for violence, as well as mental health symptoms, to ensure youth receive evidence-based, culturally competent, trauma-informed, and healing-centered mental health care.

CLINICS CARE POINTS

- Children with mental illness are much more likely to be victims of violence than perpetrators.
- Specific mental health conditions have been associated with violence and/or aggressive behaviors, although most children with these diagnoses are nonviolent.
- Children exposed to violence are at risk of developing mental health symptoms thereafter, regardless of whether exposure is direct or indirect.
- Younger children may have more internalizing symptoms following violence exposure, while adolescents may have more externalizing symptoms.
- Pediatric clinicians should practice trauma-informed care by learning about their patients' trauma exposure and associated mental health symptoms at each visit using validated tools when possible.
- For children who screen positive for mental health symptoms, pediatric clinicians should provide reassurance, simple interventions (ie, breathing exercises), and appropriate referrals to treatment.

CONFLICTS OF INTEREST DISCLOSURES

The authors have no conflicts of interest relevant to this article to disclose.

REFERENCES

1. Bitsko RH, Claussen AH, Lichstein J, et al. Mental health surveillance among children — United States, 2013–2019. MMWR Suppl 2022;71(2):1–42.
2. Whitney DG, Peterson MD. US national and state-level prevalence of mental health disorders and disparities of mental health care use in children. JAMA Pediatr 2019;173(4):389–91.
3. Centers for Disease Control and Prevention: National Center for Injury Prevention and Control. Web-based Injury Statistics Query and Reporting System (WISQARS). 2020. Available at: https://www.cdc.gov/injury/wisqars/index.html. Accessed August 9, 2021.
4. AAP-AACAP-CHA Declaration of a national emergency in child and adolescent mental health. Available at: https://www.aap.org/en/advocacy/child-and-adolescent-healthy-mental-development/aap-aacap-cha-declaration-of-a-national-emergency-in-child-and-adolescent-mental-health/. Accessed December 12, 2021.
5. Mannix R, Lee LK, Fleegler EW. Coronavirus disease 2019 (COVID-19) and firearms in the United States: will an epidemic of suicide follow? Ann Intern Med 2020;173(3):228–9.

6. Gastineau KAB, Williams DJ, Hall M, et al. Pediatric firearm-related hospital encounters during the SARS-CoV-2 Pandemic. Pediatrics 2021;148(2). https://doi.org/10.1542/peds.2021-050223.

7. Cappa C, Jijon I. COVID-19 and violence against children: a review of early studies. Child Abuse Negl 2021;116:105053.

8. De Boer C, Ghomrawi HM, Bouchard ME, et al. Effect of the COVID-19 pandemic on presentation and severity of traumatic injury due to physical child abuse across US children's hospitals. J Pediatr Surg 2022;57(4):726–31.

9. Varshney M, Mahapatra A, Krishnan V, et al. Violence and mental illness: what is the true story? J Epidemiol Community Heal 2016;70(3):223–5.

10. Hughes K, Bellis MA, Hardcastle KA, et al. The effect of multiple adverse childhood experiences on health: a systematic review and meta-analysis. Lancet Public Heal 2017;2(8):e356–66.

11. Maniglio R. Severe mental illness and criminal victimization: a systematic review. Acta Psychiatr Scand 2009;119(3):180–91.

12. Monahan J, Vesselinov R, Robbins PC, et al. Violence to others, violent self-victimization, and violent victimization by others among persons with a mental illness. Psychiatr Serv 2017;68(5):516–9.

13. Teplin LA, McClelland GM, Abram KM, et al. Crime victimization in adults with severe mental illness: comparison with the National Crime Victimization Survey. Arch Gen Psychiatry 2005;62(8):911–21.

14. Turner HA, Finkelhor D, Ormrod R. Child mental health problems as risk factors for victimization. Child Maltreat 2009;15(2):132–43.

15. Whiting D, Lichtenstein P, Fazel S. Violence and mental disorders: a structured review of associations by individual diagnoses, risk factors, and risk assessment. Lancet Psychiatr 2021;8(2):150–61.

16. Elbogen EB, Johnson SC. The intricate link between violence and mental disorder: results from the National Epidemiologic Survey on Alcohol and Related Conditions. Arch Gen Psychiatry 2009;66(2):152–61.

17. Walsh E, Buchanan A, Fahy T. Violence and schizophrenia: examining the evidence. Br J Psychiatry 2002;180:490–5.

18. Senior M, Fazel S, Tsiachristas A. The economic impact of violence perpetration in severe mental illness: a retrospective, prevalence-based analysis in England and Wales. Lancet Public Heal 2020;5(2):e99–106.

19. Connor DF. Aggression and antisocial behavior in children and adolescents: research and treatment. Guilford Press; 2002.

20. Teplin LA, Abram KM, McClelland GM, et al. Psychiatric Disorders in Youth in Juvenile Detention. Arch Gen Psychiatry 2002;59(12):1133.

21. Boots DP, Wareham J. Mental health and violent offending in Chicago youth: a multilevel approach. Office of Justice Programs; 2019. Available at: https://www.ojp.gov/ncjrs/virtual-library/abstracts/mental-health-and-violent-offending-chicago-youth-multilevel. Accessed August 26, 2022.

22. Fadus MC, Ginsburg KR, Sobowale K, et al. Unconscious bias and the diagnosis of disruptive behavior disorders and ADHD in African American and Hispanic youth. Acad Psychiatry 2020;44(1):95.

23. Simon KM. Them and me — the care and treatment of Black boys in America. N Engl J Med 2020;383(20):1904–5.

24. Connolly EJ. Further evaluating the relationship between adverse childhood experiences, antisocial behavior, and violent victimization: a sibling-comparison analysis. Youth Violence Juv Justice 2020;18(1):3–23.

25. Hodgetts S, Nicholas D, Zwaigenbaum L. Home sweet home? families' experiences with aggression in children with autism spectrum disorders. Focus Autism Other Dev Disabil 2013;28(3):166–74. https://doi.org/10.1177/1088357612472932.

26. Mazurek MO, Kanne SM, Wodka EL. Physical aggression in children and adolescents with autism spectrum disorders. Res Autism Spectr Disord 2013;7(3): 455–65.

27. Hazen EP, Ravichandran C, Hureau AR, et al. Agitation in patients with autism spectrum disorder admitted to inpatient pediatric medical units. Pediatrics 2020;145(Suppl 1):108–16.

28. Fitzpatrick SE, Srivorakiat L, Wink LK, et al. Aggression in autism spectrum disorder: presentation and treatment options. Neuropsychiatr Dis Treat 2016;12: 1525–38.

29. Barzman DH, Brackenbury L, Sonnier L, et al. Brief rating of aggression by children and adolescents (BRACHA): development of a tool for assessing risk of inpatients' aggressive behavior. J Am Acad Psychiatry Law 2011;39(2):170–9.

30. Barzman D, Mossman D, Sonnier L, et al. Brief rating of aggression by children and adolescents (BRACHA): a reliability study. J Am Acad Psychiatry Law 2012;40(3):374–82.

31. Ni Y, Barzman D, Bachtel A, et al. Finding warning markers: leveraging natural language processing and machine learning technologies to detect risk of school violence. Int J Med Inform 2020;139:104137.

32. Robinson J, Bailey E, Witt K, et al. What works in youth suicide prevention? A systematic review and meta-analysis. EClinicalMedicine 2018;4-5:52–91.

33. Hammond WR, Whitaker DJ, Lutzker JR, et al. Setting a violence prevention agenda at the centers for disease control and prevention. Aggress Violent Behav 2006;11(2):112–9.

34. Ranney M, Karb R, Ehrlich P, et al. What are the long-term consequences of youth exposure to firearm injury, and how do we prevent them? A scoping review. J Behav Med 2019;42(4):724–40.

35. LeMoult J, Humphreys KL, Tracy A, et al. Meta-analysis: exposure to early life stress and risk for depression in childhood and adolescence. J Am Acad Child Adolesc Psychiatry 2020;59(7):842–55.

36. Bancalari P, Sommer M, Rajan S. Youth exposure to endemic community gun violence: a systematic review. Adolesc Res Rev 2022;7(3):383–417.

37. Mitchell KJ, Jones LM, Turner HA, et al. Understanding the impact of seeing gun violence and hearing gunshots in public places: findings from the Youth Firearm Risk and Safety Study. J Interpers Violence 2021;36(17–18):8835–51.

38. Oddo ER, Maldonado L, Hink AB, et al. Increase in mental health diagnoses among youth with nonfatal firearm injuries. Acad Pediatr 2021;21(7):1203–8.

39. Ehrlich PF, Pulcini CD, De Souza HG, et al. Mental health care following firearm and motor vehicle-related injuries. Ann Surg 2022;276(3):463–71.

40. Zima BT, Pulcini CD, Hoffmann JA, et al. 116 Newly detected psychiatric diagnoses among medicaid-enrolled children following firearm injury. J Am Acad Child Adolesc Psychiatry 2022;61(10):S221.

41. Turner HA, Mitchell KJ, Jones LM, et al. Gun violence exposure and posttraumatic symptoms among children and youth. J Trauma Stress 2019;32(6):881–9.

42. Oddo ER, Simpson AN, Maldonado L, et al. Mental health care utilization among children and adolescents with a firearm injury. JAMA Surg 2022. https://doi.org/10.1001/jamasurg.2022.5299.

43. Pulcini CD, Goyal MK, Hall M, et al. Nonfatal firearm injuries: utilization and expenditures for children pre- and postinjury. Acad Emerg Med 2021;28(8):840–7.
44. Fleckman JM, Drury SS, Taylor CA, et al. Role of direct and indirect violence exposure on externalizing behavior in children. J Urban Heal 2016;93(3):479–92.
45. Borg BA, Rabinak CA, Marusak HA. Violence exposure and mental health consequences among urban youth. Curr Psychol 2021. https://doi.org/10.1007/s12144-021-02141-4.
46. Fowler PJ, Tompsett CJ, Braciszewski JM, et al. Community violence: a meta-analysis on the effect of exposure and mental health outcomes of children and adolescents. Dev Psychopathol 2009;21(1):227–59.
47. Cecil CAM, Viding E, Fearon P, et al. Disentangling the mental health impact of childhood abuse and neglect. Child Abus Negl 2017;63:106–19.
48. Leeb RT, Lewis T, Zolotor AJ. A review of physical and mental health consequences of child abuse and neglect and implications for practice. Am J Lifestyle Med 2011;5(5):454–68.
49. Strathearn L, Giannotti M, Mills R, et al. Long-term cognitive, psychological, and health outcomes associated with child abuse and neglect. Pediatrics 2020; 146(4). https://doi.org/10.1542/peds.2020-0438.
50. Ackard DM, Eisenberg ME, Neumark-Sztainer D. Long-term impact of adolescent dating violence on the behavioral and psychological health of male and female youth. J Pediatr 2007;151(5):476–81.
51. Wincentak K, Connolly J, Card N. Teen dating violence: a meta-analytic review of prevalence rates. Psychol Violence 2017;7(2):224–41.
52. Exner-Cortens D, Eckenrode J, Rothman E. Longitudinal associations between teen dating violence victimization and adverse health outcomes. Pediatrics 2013;131(1):71–8.
53. Olshen E, McVeigh KH, Wunsch-Hitzig RA, et al. Dating violence, sexual assault, and suicide attempts among urban teenagers. Arch Pediatr Adolesc Med 2007; 161(6):539–45.
54. Vagi KJ, O'Malley Olsen E, Basile KC, et al. Teen dating violence (physical and sexual) among US high school students. JAMA Pediatr 2015;169(5):474.
55. Choi HJ, Weston R, Temple JR. A three-step latent class analysis to identify how different patterns of teen dating violence and psychosocial factors influence mental health. J Youth Adolesc 2017;46(4):854–66.
56. Cutter-Wilson E, Richmond T. Understanding teen dating violence. Curr Opin Pediatr 2011;23(4):379–83.
57. Kitzmann KM, Gaylord NK, Holt AR, et al. Child witnesses to domestic violence: a meta-analytic review. J Consult Clin Psychol 2003;71(2):339–52.
58. Meltzer H, Doos L, Vostanis P, et al. The mental health of children who witness domestic violence. Child Fam Soc Work 2009;14(4):491–501.
59. Johnsona RM, Kotch JB, Catellier DJ, et al. Adverse behavioral and emotional outcomes from child abuse and witnessed violence. Child Maltreat 2002;7(3): 179–86.
60. Leibbrand C, Hill H, Rowhani-Rahbar A, et al. Invisible wounds: community exposure to gun homicides and adolescents' mental health and behavioral outcomes. SSM - Popul Heal 2020;12:100689.
61. Vasan A, Mitchell HK, Fein JA, et al. Association of neighborhood gun violence with mental health-related pediatric emergency department utilization. JAMA Pediatr 2021;175(12):1244–51.

62. Quimby D, Dusing CR, Deane K, et al. Gun exposure among Black American youth residing in low-income urban environments. J Black Psychol 2018;44(4): 322–46.

63. Lambert SF, Copeland-Linder N, Ialongo NS. Longitudinal associations between community violence exposure and suicidality. J Adolesc Heal 2008;43(4):380–6.

64. Martin R, Rajan S, Shareef F, et al. Racial disparities in child exposure to firearm violence before and during COVID-19. Am J Prev Med 2022;63(2):204–12.

65. Guterman NB, Hahm HC, Cameron M. Adolescent victimization and subsequent use of mental health counseling services. J Adolesc Heal 2002;30(5):336–45.

66. Finkelhor D, Turner H, LaSelva D. Receipt of behavioral health services among US children and youth with adverse childhood experiences or mental health symptoms. JAMA Netw Open 2021;4(3):e211435.

67. Schreier H, Ladakakos C, Morabito D, et al. Post-traumatic stress symptoms in children after mild to moderate pediatric trauma: a longitudinal examination of symptom prevalence, correlates, and parent-child symptom reporting. J Trauma Inj Infect Crit Care 2005;58(2):353–63.

68. Dyb G, Holen A, Brænne K, et al. Parent-child discrepancy in reporting children's post-traumatic stress reactions after a traffic accident. Nord J Psychiatry 2003; 57(5):339–44.

69. Skar A-MS, Jensen TK, Harpviken AN. Who reports what? A comparison of child and caregivers' reports of child trauma exposure and associations to post-traumatic stress symptoms and functional impairment in child and adolescent mental health clinics. Res Child Adolesc Psychopathol 2021;49(7):919–34.

70. Juillard C, Cooperman L, Allen I, et al. A decade of hospital-based violence inter-vention. J Trauma Acute Care Surg 2016;81(6):1156–61.

71. Myers RK, Vega L, Culyba AJ, et al. The psychosocial needs of adolescent males following interpersonal assault. J Adolesc Heal 2017;61(2):262–5.

72. Burkhart K, Asogwa K, Muzaffar N, et al. Pediatric integrated care models: a sys-tematic review. Clin Pediatr (Phila) 2020;59(2):148–53.

73. Bagneris JR, Noël LT, Harris R, et al. School-based interventions for post-traumatic stress among children (ages 5–11): systematic review and meta-anal-ysis. School Ment Health 2021;13(4):832–44.

74. Cummings JR, Druss BG. Racial/ethnic differences in mental health service use among adolescents with major depression. J Am Acad Child Adolesc Psychiatry 2011;50(2):160–70.

75. BURNS BJ, PHILLIPS SD, WAGNER HR, et al. Mental health need and access to mental health services by youths involved with child welfare: a national survey. J Am Acad Child Adolesc Psychiatry 2004;43(8):960–70.

76. Coker TR, Elliott MN, Kataoka S, et al. Racial/ethnic disparities in the mental health care utilization of fifth grade children. Acad Pediatr 2009;9(2):89–96.

77. Gudiño OG, Lau AS, Hough RL. Immigrant status, mental health need, and mental health service utilization among high-risk hispanic and Asian Pacific Islander youth. Child Youth Care Forum 2008;37(3):139–52.

78. Liebschutz J, Schwartz S, Hoyte J, et al. A chasm between injury and care: ex-periences of black male victims of violence. J Trauma 2010;69(6):1372.

79. Zimmerman FJ. Social and economic determinants of disparities in professional help-seeking for child mental health problems: evidence from a national sample. Health Serv Res 2005;40(5p1):1514–33.

80. Muñoz RF, Mendelson T. Toward evidence-based interventions for diverse popu-lations: the San Francisco General Hospital prevention and treatment manuals. J Consult Clin Psychol 2005;73(5):790–9.

81. Richardson LA. Seeking and obtaining mental health services: what do parents expect? Arch Psychiatr Nurs 2001;15(5):223–31.

82. Wong EC, Schell TL, Marshall GN, et al. Mental health service utilization after physical trauma. Med Care 2009;47(10):1077–83.

83. Pina AA, Polo AJ, Huey SJ. Evidence-based psychosocial interventions for ethnic minority youth: the 10-year update. J Clin Child Adolesc Psychol 2019;48(2): 179–202.

84. Metzger IW, Anderson RE, Are F, et al. Healing interpersonal and racial trauma: integrating racial socialization into trauma-focused cognitive behavioral therapy for African American youth. Child Maltreat 2021;26(1):17–27.

85. Hoffmann JA, Alegría M, Alvarez K, et al. Disparities in pediatric mental and behavioral health conditions. Pediatrics 2022;150(4).

86. Lipschitz DS, Rasmusson AM, Anyan W, et al. Clinical and functional correlates of post-traumatic stress disorder in urban adolescent girls at a primary care clinic. J Am Acad Child Adolesc Psychiatry 2000;39(9):1104–11.

87. Duffee J, Szilagyi M, Forkey H, et al. Trauma-informed care in child health systems. Pediatrics 2021;148(2). https://doi.org/10.1542/PEDS.2021-052579/ 179781.

88. Corburn J, Boggan D, Muttaqi K, et al. A healing-centered approach to preventing urban gun violence: the Advance Peace Model. Humanit Soc Sci Commun 2021;8(1):142.

89. de Arellano MAR, Lyman DR, Jobe-Shields L, et al. Trauma-focused cognitive-behavioral therapy for children and adolescents: assessing the evidence. Psychiatr Serv 2014;65(5):591–602.

90. Achenbach TM, Ruffle TM. The child behavior checklist and related forms for assessing behavioral/emotional problems and competencies. Pediatr Rev 2000; 21(8):265–71.

91. Lang JM, Connell CM. Development and validation of a brief trauma screening measure for children: the Child Trauma Screen. Psychol Trauma Theory, Res Pract Policy 2017;9(3):390–8.

92. Kaplow JB, Rolon-Arroyo B, Layne CM, et al. Validation of the UCLA PTSD Reaction Index for DSM-5: a developmentally informed assessment tool for youth. J Am Acad Child Adolesc Psychiatry 2020;59(1):186–94.

93. Foa EB, Asnaani A, Zang Y, et al. Psychometrics of the Child PTSD Symptom Scale for DSM-5 for trauma-exposed children and adolescents. J Clin Child Adolesc Psychol 2018;47(1):38–46.

94. Lieberman AF, Ghosh Ippen C, Van Horn P. Child-parent psychotherapy: 6-month follow-up of a randomized controlled trial. J Am Acad Child Adolesc Psychiatry 2006;45(8):913–8.

95. Weiner DA, Schneider A, Lyons JS. Evidence-based treatments for trauma among culturally diverse foster care youth: treatment retention and outcomes. Child Youth Serv Rev 2009;31(11):1199–205.

96. California Evidence-Based Clearinghouse for Child Welfare. Available at: www. cebc4cw.org. Accessed March 19, 2023.

Media Influences on Children and Advice for Parents to Reduce Harmful Exposure to Firearm Violence in Media

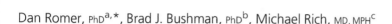

Dan Romer, PhD[a],*, Brad J. Bushman, PhD[b], Michael Rich, MD, MPH[c]

KEYWORDS

- Media violence • Firearm violence • Firearm access • Homicide • Suicide
- Mass shooting • School shooting • Neighborhood violence

KEY POINTS

- Firearm violence is a major concern for young people today, with a recent poll showing greater concern for gun violence (51%) than for abortion (47%) or climate change (37%).
- Young people learn about firearms from entertainment and social media, with movies and television cited as major sources for learning about firearms, second only to family and friends.
- Obtain a thorough media history as part of each child's psychosocial evaluation, ideally by talking directly with the child rather than through or with his or her parent(s).
- Ask children about their favorite games and movies; ask what is happening on social media (if they are on it), and ask them how they feel when watching or playing.
- Pediatricians can educate parents about those risks by sensitizing them to the potentially harmful effects of violent PG-13 movies, TV-14 dramas, and E-rated video games that involve the use of simulated firearms.

INTRODUCTION

This article examines how exposure to media violence intersects with risks that families face from firearm violence in 3 important contexts relevant to pediatricians: home, school, and neighborhood. It focuses on firearm violence because it is the most lethal

[a] Annenberg Public Policy Center, University of Pennsylvania, 202 South 36th Street, Philadelphia, PA 19104, USA; [b] School of Communication, The Ohio State University, 3016 Derby Hall, Columbus, OH 43210, USA; [c] Harvard Medical School, Digital Wellness Lab, Boston Children's Hospital, 300 Longwood Avenue, Boston, MA 02115, USA
* Corresponding author.
E-mail address: dan.romer@appc.upenn.edu

Pediatr Clin N Am 70 (2023) 1217–1224
https://doi.org/10.1016/j.pcl.2023.06.015
0031-3955/23/© 2023 Elsevier Inc. All rights reserved.

form of violence,[1] has the most direct links to influences from entertainment and social media, and is of great societal concern today. A recent report finds that firearm homicide has greatly increased since 2014 in the United States.[2] Firearms are now the number 1 cause of death in children ages 1 to 19, surpassing motor vehicle deaths.[3] Young people rank gun violence as a top concern today, and 51% report that they learn about guns from TV and movies, second behind family and friends (72%).[4]

The trend of increasing youth firearm fatalities is mirrored by increasing marketing and promotion of purchasing and using firearms for self-defense rather than for sport or hunting.[5] Some posit that the US approach to marketing is the 1 factor in contributing to much higher rates of gun injury and death than in peer countries, such as countries in Europe and Asia.[6] Also unique to the United States is the easy purchase of military style firearms, which are often used in mass shootings.[7]

As reviewed by others in this issue,[8] research over the years has documented how firearms in the home and community pose risks to health and wellbeing. Each of these risks intersects with media influences either as enhancing the use of firearms by youth or serving as means of communicating the intention to use firearms.

HOW DO MEDIA PORTRAY FIREARM VIOLENCE?

Mainstream entertainment media in movies, TV shows, and video games often feature the use of firearms, especially for virtuous purposes, such as protecting friends and family.[9–11] Each form of entertainment media has its own rating system to help parents decide what media are appropriate for their children. However, these systems suggest that adolescents ages 13+ (PG-13) can watch movies with firearms (ages 14+ for TV-14) and do not restrict consumption to those under age 17.[12,13] Even parents question whether an adolescent younger than 15 should view such portrayals,[13] and without any restrictions on those who are younger, these recommendations allow children who might not appreciate the lethality of firearms to view them as playthings.[14,15]

The portrayal of firearms in PG-13 movies has nearly tripled in the over 30 years since this specific rating was adopted.[9,11] This rating was designed to allow films with more violence and other sensitive content to be given a higher level of concern for parents than the original PG rating. However, what has happened instead is that what was formerly rated R (for ages 17+) has migrated to the PG-13 category with some adjustments to make it less upsetting to adolescents.[12] This has allowed the film industry to show more adult content to adolescents without labeling such films with the R rating that prohibits viewing for children under age 17.

Specifically, the violence that is shown in PG-13 movies is sanitized such that no blood or serious harm is displayed as a result of a gunshot wound. This is in contrast with R-rated movies, where the effects of firearm violence are more graphic and realistic. The result is that the PG-13 movies that are said to be acceptable for all adolescents ages 13 and older actually now often contain more firearm violence than R-rated movies.[9,11] The major difference is that the violence is less potentially upsetting to both parents and their children. This way of portraying violence has long been typical for broadcast TV.[16]

The rating system for TV similarly allows for portrayal of violence for adolescents ages 14 (TV-14) and older. The system for violent video games using simulated firearms (eg, first-person shooter games) is also porous, with many of the popular video games having ratings that are acceptable for teens (the E rating). The looseness and imprecision of this rating are particularly concerning given the findings from a recent meta-analysis ($N = 15,386$) that the association between exposure to violent video games and subsequent aggression peaked at ages 13 to 16 years.[17] The use of different ratings for different forms of entertainment media, with a variety of labels for different types of content, can be confusing to parents (eg, in 1 survey some parents thought "FV" meant "family viewing" when it really means "fantasy violence").[18]

HOW DO PARENTS FEEL ABOUT MOVIES WITH FIREARM VIOLENCE?

Research in which parents are shown clips of PG-13 movies with gun violence shows that parents are more likely to allow their children to view violent media, including the use of firearms, the more exposure they have to such media themselves.[19] This form of desensitization is observable in experiments in which parents are shown successive clips of violence. Their willingness to allow an adolescent to watch such violent movies increases as exposure to successive clips increases.[19]

Another factor that reduces parental concerns about firearm violence in movies is whether the violence is seen as virtuous. Many films with violent characters use firearms to protect family and friends, which is seen as more morally justified than when characters attack others for criminal purposes. In research in which parents are shown successive clips of firearm movie violence, their willingness to allow their children to watch such content is greater when it is seen as justified.[13] Nevertheless, on average, parents find these portrayals of virtuous violence to be acceptable primarily for adolescents ages 15 and older (2 years older than the rating age of 13).[13]

DO ADOLESCENTS RESPOND MORE FAVORABLY TO "VIRTUOUS" FIREARM VIOLENCE?

Early research on the effects of portrayals of screen violence showed that violence that appeared to be justified was more likely to be imitated.[20] In more recent research, adolescents and young adults have exhibited brain responses while watching movie violence that are sensitive to the justification of the violence. When the violence is seen as unjustified, it tends to trigger activation in the lateral orbital frontal cortex,[21,22] a brain region that responds to aversive events. However, another brain region located in the ventromedial prefrontal cortex responds to events that are seen as rewarding. In an experiment in which young people ages 18 to 22 were shown violent firearm movie clips that had either been rated as justified or not, brain responses in the 2 regions registered differential activation that followed the action in the clips. "Justified" violence tended to activate the ventromedial region, while unjustified violence activated the lateral orbitofrontal cortex.[23] This pattern of brain response suggests that young people with likely exposure to both kinds of films had become inured to "justified" gun violence, and less to gun violence that was seen as unjustified.

EFFECTS OF EXPOSURE TO MEDIA VIOLENCE IN THE HOME

Short-term exposure to movies with firearm violence has been found to increase interest in real guns and to playing with them in pairs of children ages 8 to 12. In 1 study, children were randomly assigned to watch a PG-rated movie clip with or without guns.[15] In another study, children played an E-rated video game with or without guns.[14] Afterwards, children in both studies were placed in a different room that contained toys and games for them to play with. The room also contained a file cabinet with real 9 mm (disabled) handguns hidden in the bottom drawer. If the children found the guns (almost all did), those exposed to media with guns engaged in more dangerous behaviors with a real gun (eg, touched it, held it, pulled the trigger, including while pointing the gun at themselves or their friend). This behavior was observed by a hidden camera. Thus, violent media pose great risks to families that have unsecured firearms in the home.

A long history of research shows that repeated exposure to violent entertainment media increases the acceptance of aggression in youth,[24] and many professional organizations warn about this influence on youth, including the American Academy of Pediatrics, the American Psychological Association, and the United Nations.[25] More recent research suggests that repeated engagement with violent video games in children and adolescents also increases risks for aggressive behavior.[26]

Heavy use of the Internet, social media and/or video games may be sign of depression and social isolation.[27–29] If a child exhibits excessive media use and withdrawal from family, friends and favorite activities, parents should seek advice from a clinical professional on whether mental health counselling is needed.

EFFECTS OF EXPOSURE TO MEDIA VIOLENCE ON RISKS IN SCHOOLS AND THE COMMUNITY

Recent research suggests that the increase in gun violence on popular TV dramas was associated with greater use of firearms in homicides among 15- to 24-year-olds over the period from 2000 to 2018.[10] This research examined the proportion of firearm use for violent purposes in TV dramas and found that this proportion increased over the study period. At the same time, the proportion of homicides involving firearms with victims in the 15- to 24-year age range also increased. This pattern suggests that viewers have seen increasing use of firearms and that this form of modeling can enhance the learning of firearm use for those with the perceived need for self-protection. This is consistent with earlier research suggesting that display of means for suicide increases the use of those means,[30] including the use of firearms, which are the deadliest means available for this purpose. In 2021, suicide accounted for most firearm deaths (56%), while homicide accounted for 44%.[31]

The normalization of guns in media increases risks for use of firearms among youth in more dangerous schools and neighborhoods where self-defense may be a greater priority. High school youths with greater exposure to violence are more likely to report more frequent carrying of weapons, including firearms.[32]

Youths may posture with firearms on social media to make themselves appear tough, as a strategy to defend against neighborhood violence.[33] Social media also can be used to threaten peers and reveal plans to engage in violence toward others in neighborhoods and schools.[34] It is also believed that social media are used by gangs to threaten violent activities toward rival factions in their neighborhood.[35] Social media and the "dark web" have become a fertile marketplace for the sale and promotion of firearms.[36] Private sellers can sell firearms on the Internet without requiring background checks.

WHAT CAN PEDIATRICIANS DO?

The pediatrician is a trusted source of information on child health and development for families. Assessment and guidance about a child's exposure to media violence and firearms are essential parts of medical histories and anticipatory guidance, and have been shown to reduce media exposure in children.[37–39] Although the guidance that a pediatrician or family physician can provide is heard and valued by parents, both media use and guns are issues on which parents will have fears, confusion, and strong, often extreme opinions. Even if their opinions may be counter to the best health advice, it is essential to maintain therapeutic rapport and trust, and convey what the science shows rather than one's own opinions or political beliefs. Providing such information allows parents to make an informed choice, while acknowledging their agency and the reality that they will make their own decisions for their family.

Include media use, particularly recreational media use, and access to firearms in standard of care medical history. Screens are ubiquitous, constantly available, and many children and adolescents now spend much of their waking hours on 1 screen or another. Ask about smartphone use, gaming, and social media use. Do not make assumptions about families' practices or behaviors at home. After each mass shooting many people who never had a gun have bought guns for self-protection rather than advocating for laws that could decrease the number of guns in the community.

ADVICE TO PARENTS

Model healthy, balanced media use at home. Adults should put their own devices away when with children. To children, it is hypocritical to ask them to stop playing a video game while adults are often noticed staring at their smartphones.

Monitor media use. Introduce devices, platforms, and applications as powerful tools when they are needed, not when children ask for them because "everyone else has one." When introducing a tool, explain explicitly how, when, and where it can be used in healthy ways, and how not to use it. Together, decide what the consequences would be if children misuse it. Although it is better that children avoid using violent video games, it is important to understand that if something is forbidden at home but available at a friend's house, they will play it there. If children download or access a specific game or Web site, recommend that a parent play with them. This helps parents understand their child's engagement with the game and offers the opportunity to stop policing and start guiding their child toward healthy pursuits.

Monitor the media that come into the home. Parents should discuss with their child why they are concerned about their use of first-person shooter games and violent media. If a child is using these forms of media to the exclusion of healthy interaction with peers and family, further assessment may be needed to determine whether depression or another mental health condition is the reason. Parents can monitor their adolescents' interactions on social media. If threats or displays of weapons are present, this could indicate that an adolescent is at risk of victimization or perpetration of violence, including self-harm or suicide. The American Academy of Child and Adolescent Psychiatry offers a practice policy and resource library on mental health and firearms.[40]

CLINICS CARE POINTS

- Obtain a thorough media history as part of each child's psychosocial evaluation, ideally by talking directly with the child rather than through or with his or her parent(s).

- Bring genuine curiosity to asking about all forms of screen media children use, including narrative movies/television series, short-form videos, games, interactive platforms, image- and text-based social networking sites. Let them teach you. They are the experts and will share everything if they hear your interest and acceptance rather than judgment.

- Ask them about their favorite games and movies, ask what is happening on social media (if they are on it), and ask them how they feel when watching or playing.

- Content matters. When they reveal use of first- or third-person shooter games, videos that feature gun violence, or platforms that viralize violent online challenges, take the opportunity to express concern about desensitization, risk-taking, and curiosity about weapons that may translate into experimentation.

- Context matters. Ask about what devices they use media on, in what settings, and with whom they use what kinds of content. If they are posturing or competing with peers, they may go farther than they otherwise might–and, if with younger siblings or friends, they may be more likely to protect them than themselves.

- Use anticipatory guidance at each age and stage to educate families about screen devices as powerful tools and all media content as educational; if they entertain themselves with violent media, the use of firearms and other weapons to harm others may be normalized both to resolve conflicts and to defend themselves against others whom they assume to have firearms.

DISCLOSURE

The authors have no conflicts to disclose.

REFERENCES

1. Spitzer SA, Pear VA, McCort CD, et al. Incidence, distribution, and lethality of firearm injuries in California from 2005 to 2015. JAMA Netw Open 2020;3(8): e2014736.
2. Goldstick JE, Carter PM, Cunningham RM. Current epidemiological trends in firearm mortality in the United States. JAMA Psychiatr 2021;78(3):241–2.
3. Goldstick JE, Cunningham RM, Carter PM. Current causes of death in children and adolescents in the United States. N Engl J Med 2022;386(20):1955–6.
4. Project Unloaded. How gun violence impacts and weights on Gen Z. Global Strategy Group; 2022. Available at: https://www.projectunloaded.org/press/new-survey-reveals-gen-z-more-worried-about-gun-violence-than-climate-change-or-access-to-abortion?emci=19f0bbbc-d49c-ed11-994c-00224832eb73&emdi=4c507342-9a9d-ed11-994c-00224832eb73&ceid=10065377. Accessed February 24, 2023.
5. Smith VM, Siegel MB, Xuan Z, et al. Broadeniing the perspective on gun violence: an examination of the firearms industry, 1990-2015. Am J Prev Med 2017;53(5): 584–91.
6. Naghavi M. Global Burden of Disease 2016 Injury Collaborators. Global mortality from firearms, 1990-2016. JAMA 2018;320(8):792–814.
7. Giffords Law Center. Assault weapons. Available at: https://giffords.org/lawcenter/gun-laws/policy-areas/hardware-ammunition/assault-weapons/. Accessed February 23, 2023.
8. Gastineau KAB, McKay S. Firearm injury prevention. Pediatr Clin North Am.
9. Bushman BJ, Jamieson PE, Weitz I, et al. Gun violence trends in movies. Pediatrics 2013;132(6):1014–8.
10. Jamieson PE, Romer D. The association between the use of gun violence in popular US primetime television dramas and homicides attributable to firearms, 2000-2018. PLoS One 2021;16(3):e0247780.
11. Romer D, Jamieson PE, Jamieson KH. The continuing rise of gun violence in PG-13 movies, 1985-2015. Pediatrics 2017;139(2):e20162891.
12. Nalkur PG, Jamieson PE, Romer D. The effectiveness of the Motion Picture Association of America's rating system in screening explicit violence and sex in top-grossing movies from 1950 to 2006. J Adolesc Health 2010;47(5):440–7.
13. Romer D, Jamieson PE, Jamieson KH, et al. Parental desensitization to gun violence in PG-13 movies. Pediatrics 2018;141(6):e20173491.

14. Chang JH, Bushman BJ. Effect of exposure to gun violence in video games on children's dangerous behavior with real guns: a randomized clinical trial. JAMA Netw Open 2019;2(5):e194319.

15. Dillon KP, Bushman BJ. Deadly child's play: exposure to gun violence in movies increases interest in real guns. JAMA Pediatr 2017. https://doi.org/10.1001/jamapediatrics.2017.2229.

16. Potter WJ. Adolescents and television violence. In: Jamieson PE, Romer D, editors. *The changing portrayal of adolescents in the media since 1950*. New York: Oxford University Press; 2008. p. 221–49.

17. Burkhardt J, Lenhard WA. Meta-analysis on the longitudinal, age-dependent effects of violent video games on aggression. Media Psychol 2022;25(3):499–512.

18. Rideout V. Parents, children & media: A Kaiser Family Foundation survey. The Henry J. Kaiser Foundation; 2007. p. 4. Available at: https://www.kff.org/other/poll-finding/parents-children-media-a-kaiser-family-foundation/. Accessed July 25, 2023.

19. Romer D, Jamieson PE, Bushman BJ, et al. Parental desensitization to violence and sex in movies. Pediatrics 2014;134:877–84.

20. Berkowitz L. Some effects of thoughts on anti- and prosocial influences of media events: a cognitive-neoassociation analysis. J Pers Soc Psychol 1984;95(3):410–27.

21. Alia-Klein N, Wang GJ, Preston-Campbell RN, et al. Reactions to media violence: it's in the brain of the beholder. PLoS One 2014;9(9):e107260.

22. Kelly CR, Grinband J, Hirsch J. Repeated exposure to media violence is associated with diminished response in an inhibitory frontolimbic network. PLoS One 2012;2(12):e1268.

23. Adebimpe A, Bassett DS, Jamieson PE, et al. Intersubject synchronization of late adolescent brain responses to violent movies: a virtue-ethics approach. Front Behav Neurosci 2019;13(260):1–13.

24. Anderson CA, Bushman BJ, Bartholow BD, et al. Screen violence and youth behavior. Pediatrics 2017;140(s2):e20161758.

25. Bushman B.J. Statements on media violence by major scientific groups. 2023. Available at: https://u.osu.edu/bushman.20/statements-on-media-violence-effects-by-major-scientific-groups/ . Accessed July 25, 2023.

26. Teng Z, Nie Q, Guo C, et al. A longitudinal study of link between exposure to violent video games and aggression in Chinese adolescents: The mediating role of moral disengagement. Dev Psychobiol 2019;55(1):184–95.

27. Romer D, Bagdasarov Z, More E. Older versus newer media and the well-being of United States youth: results from a national longitudinal panel. J Adolesc Health 2013;52:613–9.

28. Bleakley A, Ellithorpe ME, Romer D. The role of parents in problematic internet use among adolescents. Media Commun 2016;4(3):24–34.

29. Kaess M, Klar J, Kindler J, et al. Excessive and pathological internet use–risk behavior or psychopathology? Addict Behav 2021;123:107045.

30. Stack S. Contributing factors to suicide: political, social, cultural and economic. Prev Med 2021;152:1–13.

31. Simon TR, Kegler SR, Zwald ML, et al. Increase in firearm homicide and suicide rates–United States, 2020-2021. MMWR (Morb Mortal Wkly Rep) 2022;71(40):1286–7.

32. David-Ferdon C, Clayton HB, Dahlberg LL, et al. Vital signs: prevalence of multiple forms of violence and increased health risk behaviors and conditions among youths–United States, 2019. MMWR Morb Mortal Wkly Rep 2021;70(5):167–73.

33. Stewart F. Code of the tweet: urban gang violence in the social media age. Soc Probl 2019. https://doi.org/10.1093/socpro/spz010.

34. Patton DU, Leonard P, Elaesser C, et al. What's a threat on social media? How Black and Latino Chicago young men define and navigate threats online. Youth Soc 2019;51(6):756–72.

35. Patton DU, Eschmann RD, Elsaesser C, et al. Sticks, stones and Facebook accounts: what violence outreach workers know about social media and urban-based gang violence in Chicago. Comput Hum Behav 2016;65:591–600.

36. Ranney ML, Conrey FR, Perkinson L, et al. How Americans encounter guns: mixed methods content analysis of YouTube and internet search data. Prev Med 2022;165:107258.

37. American Academy of Pediatrics. Policy statement–media violence. Pedatrics 2009;124(5):1495–505.

38. Lee LK, Fleeger EW, Goyal MK, et al. Firearm-related injuries and deaths in children and youth: Injury prevention and harm reduction. Pediatrics 2022;150(6). e2022060070.

39. Barkin SL, Finch SA, Ip EH, et al. Is office-based counseling about media use, timeouts, and firearm storage effective? Results from a cluster-randomized, controlled trial. Pediatrics 2008;122(1):e15–25.

40. American Academy of Child & Adolescent Psychiatry. Policy statement on children and guns. 2022. Available at: https://www.aacap.org/AACAP/Policy_Statements/2022/Children_and_Guns.aspx . Accessed February 23, 2023.

Violence Prevention in Pediatrics
Advocacy and Legislation

Alison J. Culyba, MD, PhD, MPH[a],*, Eric W. Fleegler, MD, MPH[b],
Abdullah H. Pratt, MD[c], Lois K. Lee, MD, MPH[b]

KEYWORDS

- Advocacy • Legislation • Community partnerships • Youth violence prevention

KEY POINTS

- Pediatric clinicians have an important role in advocating for youth victims of violence, youth at risk for engagement in violence, and marginalized communities disproportionately impacted by violence.
- Prioritizing equity must be central to youth violence prevention advocacy.
- Successful advocacy requires engaging, collaborating, and partnering with individuals, clinical systems, and communities to build, study, and promote innovative and effective interventions.
- Pediatric clinicians can also engage in legislative advocacy for policies, regulations, and legislation to address the social determinants of health as well as firearm and violence prevention at the institutional, local, state, and national levels.

INTRODUCTION

Pediatric clinicians have a natural role in advocating for issues to advance and promote the health of children and adolescents in their care. There are several strategies that can be adopted to advance advocacy goals and used across a range of practice settings.[1] These strategies include (1) education of patients and caregivers, health care professionals, researchers, and the lay community; (2) community engagement; and (3) advocacy for policy or regulatory change at the institutional, local, state, and national levels (**Table 1**).[1] Because youth violence disproportionately affects marginalized communities, advocacy efforts should additionally focus on addressing the structural inequities and health disparities affecting these youth.[2–4]

a Division of Adolescent and Young Adult Medicine, UPMC Children's Hospital of Pittsburgh, University of Pittsburgh School of Medicine, 120 Lytton Avenue, Suite 302, Pittsburgh, PA 15217, USA; b Division of Emergency Medicine, Boston Children's Hospital, 300 Longwood Avenue, Boston, MA 02115, USA; c Section of Emergency Medicine, The University of Chicago Medical Center, 5841 South Maryland Avenue, Chicago, IL 60637, USA
* Corresponding author.
E-mail address: alison.culyba@chp.edu

Pediatr Clin N Am 70 (2023) 1225–1238
https://doi.org/10.1016/j.pcl.2023.06.012
0031-3955/23/© 2023 Elsevier Inc. All rights reserved.

		Policy and Regulatory
Education	**Community Engagement**	**Change**
Institutional	Institutional	Institutional

• Formal lectures to medical audience
• Provide advocacy opportunities to trainees
	• Develop and/or advance partnerships between institutions and communities for youth violence prevention and intervention programs
	• Partner with communities to advocate for resources to create safer neighborhood spaces for children and youth
		• Develop policies and procedures to provide trauma-informed care for youth victims of violence
		• Work with professional organizations (eg, AAP) or institution for opportunities to engage with policymakers
		• Provide resources to address social determinants of health for youth patients
		  ○ Medical-financial partnerships
		  ○ Food insecurity
		  ○ Housing insecurity
		  ○ Social needs
		  ○ Connection to social programs

Community	Community	Community
• Community-based audience • Law enforcement • Media, including social media	• Engage with community-based violence prevention organizations	• Partner with schools and community organizations to support youth violence intervention and prevention programs
Policy	Policy	Policy
• Provide education for policy makers and their staff	• Partner with medical societies for support with legislative advocacy	• Provide oral or written testimony for policies and legislation supporting youth violence prevention and intervention

Table 1
Advocacy strategies to address youth violence

Adapted from Beers LS, Williams-Willingham MA, Chamberlain LJ. Making advocacy part of your job. Pediatr Clin North Am 2023;70:25–34.

Given the complexities of youth violence prevention, advocacy must support all aspects of a public health approach focused on prevention, intervention, and restoration. Advocacy related to youth violence prevention should encompass 3 interlinked groups (**Fig. 1**):[5]

- Group one: youth victims of, and witnesses to, violence
- Group two: youth at risk for engagement in violence
- Group three: marginalized communities disproportionately impacted by violence

Group one focuses on individual *youth victims of, and witnesses to, violence*. Advocacy can focus on addressing acute and long-term physical, behavioral, and mental health consequences as well as prevention of future violence among violently injured patients. After the acute event and/or injury, this begins with the provision of healing-centered care, which includes recognition of the signs and symptoms of trauma,

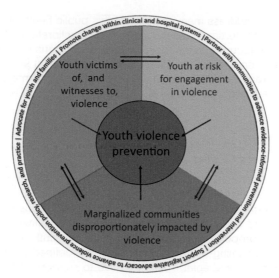

Fig. 1. Role of pediatric clinicians in advocacy related to youth violence prevention. (*Adapted from* Richmond, Kotelchuk, "The Effects of Political Process on the Delivery of Health Services," in Handbook of Health Professions Education, ed. McGuire and others (1983).)

avoidance of retraumatization, and development of appropriate policies and procedures for healing-centered patient care.[6] For restoration after violence has occurred, advocacy also includes the facilitation of patients' and families' access to services for physical and mental health, substance abuse treatment, and hospital- and community-based violence intervention and prevention programs.[5]

Group two focuses on *youth at risk for engagement in violence*. Here, advocacy can focus on policies to decrease youth firearm access,[7] improve access to resources for mental health care, and provide supervision and mentorship for youth. Advocacy should include the support and promotion of school- and community-based violence intervention and prevention programs for youth at risk for engagement in violence. Types of interventions may include after-school programs and evening and weekend activities, mentorship from trusted adults, and job opportunities (during both the school year and summer breaks).[8–11]

Group three focuses on *interventions for marginalized communities disproportionately impacted by violence*. At the larger community level, advocacy should focus on addressing sociostructural inequities that underpin violence. These inequities may include, but are not limited to, safe housing, education and job opportunities, enhancement of the school environment and safe spaces for youth to spend time, education of law enforcement in restorative justice practices, and community-engaged neighborhood improvement, including the greening and rehabilitation of vacant spaces.[12–15] In addition, it is important to advocate for policies and funding to support critical incident response and hot spot mediation to prevent future violence.[13] Advocacy for community interventions can include legislative advocacy for policies, regulations, and legislation to address the social determinants of health as well as firearm and violence prevention—this type of legislative advocacy may occur at the local, state, and national levels.[16,17]

Advocacy by pediatric clinicians provides a critical voice to represent youth in their care to address the myriad contributors and effects of youth violence (see **Table 1**). Institutional, community, state, and federal programs, as well as policies and legislation can help support and address many aspects of this public health approach with primary, secondary, and tertiary prevention for the amelioration of youth violence (**Table 2**). This article focuses on the role of pediatric clinicians in advocacy for youth and families, promotion of change within clinical and hospital systems, partnership with communities to advance evidence-informed prevention and intervention, and support of legislative advocacy to advance violence prevention policy, research, and practice.

DISCUSSION
Advocate for Youth and Families

Youth violence results from a complex interplay of factors across multiple levels of the social ecology.[18] Prevention of violence and mitigation of the consequences of violence require addressing the root causes. These root causes include racism, poverty, historical and current structural oppression, and disinvestment in communities, all of which disproportionately impact marginalized youth and families. The creation of inclusive and healing-centered clinical spaces, defined as spaces promoting cohesion of mind, body, and spirit,[19] is imperative to support a holistic approach to fostering well-being among youth and families impacted by violence—one that centers on culture, civic action, and collective healing.[20] Youth injured or impacted by violence can experience medical needs, mental health needs, and health-related social needs (eg, financial needs, transportation needs, assistance with connection to community programs). Clinicians should routinely assess individualized needs and work with families to provide linkage to services. In some instances, letters of medical necessity and direct advocacy with school systems are necessary to advocate for youth in the aftermath of violence and to manage safety concerns. Clinicians should be attuned to the broader ripple effects of violence across communities and connect youth with trauma-informed mental health services when indicated.

Promote Change Within Clinical and Hospital Systems

Clinicians can advocate for hospital support for programs that address violence prevention. One example includes the distribution of safer storage devices for firearms through clinical settings, which research has demonstrated can improve rates of safer storage.[21] Work with hospitals to identify funding for firearm safer storage devices can expand access to this harm reduction strategy for youth and families.

Clinicians can also play a vital role in advocacy for hospital support for tertiary prevention programs designed to meet the needs of violently injured youth. Hospital-based violence intervention programs (HVIPs) are interdisciplinary programs that provide case management and linkage to services for youth and families in the aftermath of violence to promote healing and recovery. These programs have been shown to reduce reinjury and future violence involvement.[22] Although HVIPs begin in hospital settings, their role extends beyond clinical spaces to foster community-based case management and linkage to services. Clinicians serve as key points of contact and interface between the health care and community systems. As trusted care providers, clinicians can share their clinical expertise to ensure that HVIPs and related programs are designed to meet the unique needs of their patients and local communities. Critical to this work is the establishment of strong connections with community organizations that support youth and families, which includes victim service agencies and community-based violence prevention programs. Clinicians can advocate for the implementation of these programs, as well as for dedicated funding from hospitals and health systems to support collaboration between community-based programs.

Table 2
Primary, secondary, and tertiary prevention strategies to prevent youth violence

Primary Prevention Community	Secondary Prevention Youth at Risk	Tertiary Prevention Youth Victim
Institutional • Improve access to physical and mental health services • Universal firearm safety counseling and provision of safer storage devices	Institutional • Hospital-based violence *prevention* programs • Hospital-based violence *intervention* programs	Institutional • Provide trauma-informed care • Access services for physical and mental health and substance abuse treatment • Hospital-based violence intervention programs
Community • Safe housing • Safe and supportive school environment • School and after-school programs for youth • Law enforcement education • Neighborhood improvement of spaces	Community • School- and community-based violence *prevention* programs • School- and community-based violence *intervention* programs • Mentorship programs • Sports programs • Job training and opportunities	Community • Linkage to community-based resources • Violence interruption programs to mediate conflicts and reduce retaliation • Community-based programs to support coping and recovery
Policy Address: • Social determinants of health • Antipoverty policies Develop: • Firearm injury prevention • Resources for violence prevention programs and research	Policy • Decrease firearm access among youth • Resources for critical incident response • Resources for hot spot mediation • Resources for violence prevention programs and research	Policy • Funding for victims' assistance • Funding for emergency basic needs • Resources for housing relocation to address acute safety concerns

Partner with Communities to Advance Evidence-Informed Prevention and Intervention

As youth-serving professionals, pediatric clinicians can enhance their impact by expanding beyond clinical encounters to the development of partnerships with communities. The Health Alliance for Violence Intervention (HAVI) is leading national efforts to build a violence prevention ecosystem through "comprehensive, community-based strategies that link various proven public health tools—such as outreach, the violence reduction strategy, hospital-based violence intervention programs, and/or trauma-informed care—to essential supports and services" (thehavi.org). The HAVI is applying an integrated approach **(Fig. 2)** with city-specific guidance available (https://www.cviecosystem.org). As communities seek to grow these services, pediatric clinicians can provide critical advocacy for implementation of these evidence-informed models, with a focus on the unique developmental needs of youth. Pediatric clinicians can seek opportunities to inform or directly contribute to evaluation of programs to ensure they are meeting the needs of youth and families.

Pediatric clinicians can also play an important role in advocating for safe, supportive, and inclusive school environments. Although school shootings comprise a small percent of the overall burden of youth violence and firearm-related violence, they often catalyze conversations at the local and national levels. There is little evidence to support the claim that arming teachers or increasing security presence on school campuses improves student safety; instead, these approaches may cause harm.[23] The Department of Education and the US Secret Service recommend the Safe Schools

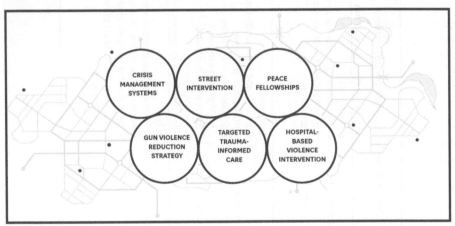

Fig. 2. Community violence intervention ecosystem. *Crisis management systems*: Deploy street outreach workers who mediate conflicts and connect individuals to wraparound services. *Street outreach*: Deploy street outreach workers to prevent violence, provide crisis response, and connect individuals to community resources. *Peace fellowships*: Deploy street outreach workers to intervene in violence and enrol participants in a longitudinal program that includes mentoring, community support and services, peer fellowship, and stipends. *Gun violence reduction strategy*: Use data-driven identification of people and groups at highest risk for firearm violence and provide intensive services, supports, and opportunities. *Targeted trauma-informed care*: Conduct outreach to provide trauma-informed comprehensive physical, mental, and psychosocial care. *Hospital-based violence intervention*: Connect with victims following violent injury and provide trauma-informed, community-based resources and case management to promote healing. (Adapted with permission from the Health Alliance for Violence Intervention CVI Ecosystem Model, 2023.)

Initiative, which focuses on developing the capacity to evaluate and respond to potential school violence threats alongside developing positive school environments, fostering social-emotional competence, and connecting youth at risk for involvement with violence prevention services.[24] Safe Communities Safe Schools provides a roadmap for tailored assessment and intervention.[25] Clinicians familiar with these recommendations can offer evidence-informed guidance to local school districts to inform policies and practices.

Universal violence prevention programs focused on positive youth development and bullying prevention delivered in school settings are also essential to improve safety and reduce youth violence.[25] Blueprints for Healthy Youth Development provides a registry of evidence-based prevention programs implemented at the family, school, and community levels (https://www.blueprintsprograms.org/). This registry can serve as a resource for clinicians who work in partnership with communities to identify and implement violence prevention programs. Programs that strengthen peer and adolescent-adult relationships and foster antiviolence social norms can be particularly impactful.[26,27] As trusted sources of information on pediatric health, pediatric clinicians can play an instrumental role in advocacy for the implementation of programs supported by the best scientific evidence. Academic-community partnerships grounded in equity and reciprocity are also important in the evaluation of program effectiveness across diverse settings, which should contribute to the evidence base.[28]

A growing body of scholarship also demonstrates the importance of community-level interventions to improve safety and reduce violence.[29] Community-level programs, such as Crime Prevention Through Environmental Design, which change the physical environment of a neighborhood by investing in community spaces (eg, greening abandoned lots and remediating blighted properties), can decrease community violence.[29–31] As these types of interventions are implemented across the United States, clinicians can advocate for a focus on equity and pediatric health outcomes as integral components of implementation and evaluation. Clinicians connected with youth-serving organizations are well-positioned to bring interdisciplinary groups together in service of a shared goal to reduce youth violence.

Legislative Advocacy to Advance Violence Prevention Policy, Research, and Practice

Pediatric clinicians have the experience and credibility to couple clinical experiences with research evidence to guide legislative recommendations. Because firearms are important drivers of violence-related morbidity and mortality, advocacy for evidence-informed firearm safety legislation at the state and federal levels is an important component of a comprehensive legislative approach to violence prevention. Stronger firearm safety laws are associated with lower rates of firearm homicide.[32–35] Evidence-informed policies include universal background checks, permit to purchase a firearm, child access prevention laws, intimate partner violence-related firearm laws, and extreme risk protection orders ([ERPO] or "red flag laws").[36–38]

At the national level, the Bipartisan Safer Communities Act, signed into law on June 25, 2022, represents an important advancement in firearm safety and violence prevention. Many health organizations, including the American Academy of Pediatrics (AAP), played an instrumental role in the bill's passage. More than 300 pediatricians contributed testimonies submitted to the congressional record.[39] The bill includes funding for the creation and administration of state ERPO, also known as red flag laws; expands prohibitions of gun ownership related to domestic violence; clarifies the definition of federally-licensed firearm dealers to expand sellers who are required to conduct background checks; increases the review process for sales to individuals younger than

21 years; and provides funding for community-based violence prevention initiatives. The law also enlarges mental health service programs and school-based supports to foster safer school environments and address bullying, violence, and hate in school settings.[40]

Historically, funding for clinical and community-based violence prevention and intervention programming has been limited, with programs forced to piece together grant and philanthropic funds to support their work. Although the past decade has seen an increase in firearm safety and violence prevention research, funding to advance the science remains disproportionately low compared with the scope of the problem. Per one pediatric death, funding from 2008 to 2017 for firearms was $537, compared with $25 million for HIV, $26,136 for motor vehicle crashes, and $195,508 for cancer.[41] From 2004 to 2014, compared with other leading causes of death, firearm violence received only 1.6% of predicted research funding, although federal funding to the Centers for Disease Control and Prevention (CDC) and National Institutes of Health (NIH) increased as of 2020.[42] More recently, there has been increased recognition of the critical importance of these programs to support the health and well-being of youth and families. Legislation such as the Bipartisan Solutions to Cyclical Violence Act[43] and state Medicaid bills to fund the work of violence prevention professionals offer new avenues to integrate violence prevention within the health landscape. Pediatric clinicians can play an important role in advocating for these laws at the state and federal levels.

There are specific opportunities for pediatricians to develop advocacy skills, including the Trainees for Injury Prevention program led by the Center for Injury Research and Policy at Nationwide Children's Hospital and sponsored by the AAP. This year-long program provides didactic and experiential learning for medical students, residents, and fellows in a broad range of injury advocacy topics and culminates in a day of action (https://www.nationwidechildrens.org/research/areas-of-research/center-for-injury-research-and-policy/education-and-training/t4cip). For pediatric clinicians working in an academic setting, the Academic Pediatric Association's Health Policy Scholars Program is a three-year career development program for faculty interested in learning how to apply a scholarly approach to child health advocacy. In addition, the AAP Annual Advocacy Conference offers advocacy skills-building workshops, opportunities to engage with leaders, and hands-on experience meeting with legislators to advance a pediatric health advocacy objective.

In addition to formal training opportunities, pediatricians are at times provided with unanticipated opportunities to advocate. In the wake of the mass shooting at Robb Elementary School in Uvalde, TX, USA, on May 24, 2022, Dr Roy Guerrero, the sole pediatrician in Uvalde, offered powerful testimony in the House Committee on Oversight and Reform. He reflected, "I was called here today as a witness. But I showed up because I am a doctor. Because how many years ago I swore an oath–an oath to do no harm. After witnessing firsthand, the carnage in my hometown of Uvalde, to stay silent would have betrayed that oath. Inaction is harm. Passivity is harm. Delay is harm."[44] As youth-serving professionals, we have the opportunity to advocate for the services that youth and families deserve, and also to offer our expertise in service of broader prevention approaches at the hospital and community levels.

Examples of Advocacy at the Individual and Clinical Levels

In attempts to address factors leading to the growing rate of violent deaths faced by youth in the South Side of Chicago, Dr Abdullah Hasan Pratt has developed and implemented 3 evidence-based initiatives informed by his lived experience growing up in this area coupled by his professional experience as an emergency medicine physician at the University of Chicago. In 2018, in response to a lack of resources dedicated toward lay bystander training of hemorrhage control tactics in communities experiencing nation-leading rates of gun violence, Dr Pratt initiated the Medical Careers Exposure and Emergency Preparedness Program (MedCEEP). Through Stop the Bleed (STB) workshops in schools surrounding The University of Chicago's Level One Trauma Center, his team of medical students, residents, nurses, and emergency medical technicians have trained more than 7000 local youth.

In addition, to respond to the students' desire to process their firsthand experiences witnessing gun violence, Dr Pratt developed the Trauma Recovery and Prevention of Violence Program (TRAP Violence). Through student-led and facilitator-guided (Violence Recovery Specialists and trauma behavioral health professional) workshops, TRAP Violence aims to increase students' awareness of the factors that lead to violence, improve trauma coping skills, develop conflict resolution skills, and provide mental health awareness to recognize and respond to potentially violent encounters. Also, based on literature supporting the protective effects of contact youth sports programs (eg, youth football, boxing, martial arts, and basketball), Dr Pratt and his team have a third program focusing on improving the safety of high-impact sports. The team has provided more than 1000 free sports physicals and attended more than 100 events as sideline/ringside physician.

For staffing, these programs rely on volunteers and the programs' utility as educational opportunities for trainees interested in careers in public health, health policy, Emergency Medical Services (EMS), and sports medicine. However, implementation of low-cost programs relying on the donated time and services of medical students, residents, attending physicians, and other clinical staff members who have unpredictable schedules due to the demanding nature of their jobs poses many challenges. The current funding structure of Dr Pratt's volunteer-based workforce creates conflict for those who must choose between reporting to work to earn wages for their families and coming to these sessions without financial compensation. As a result, although each volunteer is dedicated to the mission of reducing violence, there is a possibility of fatigue among those who deliver the program content. Many of these challenges could be substantially mitigated with adequate funding, which includes honorariums for presenters, administrative and research support, and buy-down for faculty member effort. Significant support is required to ensure comprehensive violence prevention programs are equitably dispersed in communities that experience the highest rates of violence but often have the fewest resources to address its root causes. Clinicians can play a critical role in advocating for the development and financial sustainability of these programs.

Example of Advocacy at the Hospital Level

At the hospital level, an adolescent medicine physician, a pediatric trauma surgeon, and a social worker partnered to develop an HVIP integrated within an adolescent medical home at the UPMC Children's Hospital of Pittsburgh. The team worked together to identify existing resources within the health system and to secure support from leadership and local philanthropic organizations to launch the Empowering Teens to Thrive program. Through a quality improvement framework, they refined the referral, outreach, and intervention components to meet the needs of injured youth. The team gathered metrics about the services they provided, client outcomes, and unmet needs, which supported grant applications to grow the program; they explored reimbursement models to increase financial sustainability. The program was awarded funding from the Allegheny County Health Department Office of Violence

Prevention, the Substance Abuse and Mental Health Services Administration (SAMHSA), and the Pennsylvania Commission on Crime and Delinquency. This program is now integrated into the health system and provides individualized services to youth and families to support coping and recovery (https://www.chp.edu/our-services/aya-medicine/empowering-teens-to-thrive).

Example of Advocacy at the Federal Level

On a federal level, one example of advocacy for youth violence prevention is the AAP formation of the Gun Violence Prevention (GVP) Research Roundtable Coalition. This coalition focuses on advocacy for increasing federal funding for firearm-related research, which includes funding for studies of violence intervention and prevention programs. After the Dickey amendment was passed in 1996, federal funding first for the CDC and then in 2011 for the NIH became effectively nonexistent.[45] Then in 2019 Congress appropriated $25 million for federal research funding, equally divided between the CDC and the NIH.[46] However, this funding has remained flat at $25 million in 2020, 2021, and 2022. To help Congress develop a deeper understanding of the importance of increasing funding for firearm violence research, the multidisciplinary members of the GVP Research Roundtable Coalition and its Advisory Board continue to educate congressional members about this issue.[47] Ongoing advocacy will be essential to increase funding not only for research but also for community violence intervention and prevention programs as well as policies to support the social determinants of health to address root causes of violence at the community level.

SUMMARY

Violence among children and youth can have longstanding physical, mental health, and social consequences, and long-term repercussions for families and communities. Because firearms, including firearm homicide, are the leading cause of death in US children and youth,[48] pediatric clinicians have an important role in advocacy at the individual patient, institutional, community, and policy levels to advance youth violence prevention.[1] The prioritization of equity, especially for marginalized communities in which community violence often has a higher prevalence, must be central to youth violence prevention advocacy.[17,49]

For the success of any type of advocacy, engagement, collaboration, and partnership with individuals and the community to build, study, and promote innovative and effective interventions is crucial; this includes work with community and other professional organizations, like the HAVI. The use of available resources for training and advocacy opportunities through professional organizations like the AAP can also be helpful in advancing advocacy work. Development of relationships and building partnerships with diverse stakeholders at the institutional, community, and state and federal levels is a vital part of youth violence advocacy efforts. Coalition building to bring invested stakeholders together, centered on the involved community, is a critical part of this advocacy strategy.[50,51] Work with media can also garner attention to important advocacy issues related to youth violence prevention[17] and help disseminate research to inform policy and practice.[52] This work can include publication of Op-Eds in the lay press and commentaries in peer-reviewed medical journals, and engagement in social media and other media outlets (eg, newspapers, television news, podcast).[53]

Legislative testimony, written or verbal, is another valuable type of advocacy. Pediatric clinicians have unique insight into patients and families who have experienced or are experiencing violence at the individual and/or community level and can help to amplify their message. Their lived experiences and voices as the legislator's constituent are especially important when engaging legislators and their staff around policy at the state or federal level[54]; this ensures that advocacy is focused on those most affected by youth violence. Clinicians can partner with patients and families to help bring this vital voice to policymakers for advocacy for resources for programs and research for youth violence prevention. Pediatric clinicians can share these important perspectives from their clinical experiences, while always ensuring patient confidentiality, or with permission from the patient and/or family, if confidentiality cannot be assured.[53] Clinicians can also help bring the scientific research and data on evidence-based best practices to policymakers and build relationships with them, because it is often necessary to build on advocacy efforts over time.[17]

SUMMARY

Pediatric clinicians have an important role in advocacy for youth victims of violence, youth at risk for engagement in violence, and marginalized communities disproportionately impacted by violence. Given longstanding violence inequities in which youth from marginalized communities bear a disproportionate burden of violence, equity must be central to youth violence prevention advocacy. Pediatric clinicians should work to create inclusive and healing-centered clinical spaces and support provision of trauma-informed care and linkage to clinical and community-based services for youth and families impacted by violence. Successful advocacy requires engaging, collaborating, and partnering with individuals, clinical systems, and communities to build, study, and promote innovative and effective interventions. Pediatric clinicians are ideally positioned to engage in advocacy for policies, regulations, and legislation to address the social determinants of health as well as firearm and violence prevention at the institutional, local, state, and national levels.

CLINICS CARE POINTS

- Pediatric clinicians have an important role in advocacy for youth victims of violence, youth at risk for engagement in violence, and marginalized communities disproportionately impacted by violence.

- Pediatric clinicians should work to create inclusive and healing-centered clinical spaces to support the needs of youth and families impacted by violence.

- Individual-level advocacy can occur in daily practice to promote physical and mental health of youth impacted by violence through provision of trauma-informed care and linkage to clinical and community-based services.

- Clinicians serve an important role in interdisciplinary programs by serving as a key point of contact and interface between the health care and community systems.

- Pediatric clinicians are well-positioned to couple clinical experiences with research evidence to contribute to legislative testimony and to guide policy and legislative recommendations.

DISCLOSURE

Dr E.W. Fleegler and Dr L.K. Lee receive royalties as editors for the book, "Pediatric Firearm Injuries and Fatalities: The Clinician's Guide to Policies and Approaches to Firearm Harm Prevention."

REFERENCES

1. Beers LS, Williams-Willingham MA, Chamberlain LJ. Making Advocacy Part of Your Job: Working for Children in Any Practice Setting. Pediatr Clin North Am 2023;70(1):25–34.

2. Rees CA, Monuteaux MC, Steidley I, et al. Trends and Disparities in Firearm Fatalities in the United States, 1990-2021. JAMA Netw Open 2022;5(11):e2244221.

3. Hoffmann JA, Farrell CA, Monuteaux MC, et al. Association of Pediatric Suicide With County-Level Poverty in the United States, 2007-2016. JAMA Pediatr 2020;174(3):287–94.

4. Barrett JT, Lee LK, Monuteaux MC, et al. Association of County-Level Poverty and Inequities With Firearm-Related Mortality in US Youth. JAMA Pediatr 2022;176(2): e214822.

5. Sood AB, Berkowitz SJ. Prevention of Youth Violence. A Public Health Approach. Child Adolesc Psychiatr Clin N Am 2016;25(2):243–56.

6. Fischer KR, Bakes KM, Corbin TJ, et al. Trauma-Informed Care for Violently Injured Patients in the Emergency Department. Ann Emerg Med 2019;73(2): 193–202.

7. Lee LK, Fleegler EW, Goyal MK, et al. Firearm-Related Injuries and Deaths in Children and Youth. Pediatrics 2022;150(6):1–22.

8. Bilchik S. 1999 National Report Series Juvenile Justice Bulletin; 1999. Available at: https://ojjdp.ojp.gov/library/publications/juvenile-offenders-and-victims-1999-national-report. Accessed March 1, 2023.

9. Gottfredson D.C., Gerstenblith S.A., Soulé D.A., et al., Do After School Programs Reduce Delinquency? Vol 5.; 2004. Available at: http://www.ed.gov/21stcclc. Accessed March 1, 2023.

10. Heller SB. Summer jobs reduce2 violence among disadvantaged youth. Science (1979) 2014;346(6214):1219–23.

11. Heller S., Pollack H., Davis J.M., et al., The effects of summer jobs on youth violence. Available at: https://ojjdp.ojp.gov/library/publications/effects-summer-jobs-youth-violence. Accessed March 1, 2023.

12. David-Ferndon C., Vivolo-Kantor A.M., Dahlberg L., et al., A comprehensive technical package for the prevention of youth violence and associated risk behaviors, 2016, National Center for Injury Prevention and Control, Centers for Disease Control and Prevention, Available at: https://stacks.cdc.gov/view/cdc/43085. Accessed March 1, 2023.

13. Abt TP. Towards a framework for preventing community violence among youth. Psychol Health Med 2017;22:266–85.

14. Moyer R, MacDonald JM, Ridgeway G, et al. Effect of remediating blighted vacant land on shootings: A citywide cluster randomized trial. Am J Public Health 2019;109(1):140–4.

15. Kondo MC, South EC, Branas CC, et al. The Association between Urban Tree Cover and Gun Assault: A Case-Control and Case-Crossover Study. Am J Epidemiol 2017;186(3):289–96.

16. Lee LK, Fleegler EW, Goyal MK, et al. Firearm-Related Injuries and Deaths in Children and Youth: Injury Prevention and Harm Reduction. Pediatrics 2022;150(6). https://doi.org/10.1542/peds.2022-060070.

17. Behrens D, Haasz M, Dodington J, et al. Firearm Injury Prevention Advocacy: Lessons Learned and Future Directions. Pediatr Clin North Am 2023;70(1):67–82.

18. Nation M, Chapman DA, Edmonds T, et al. Social and Structural Determinants of Health and Youth Violence: Shifting the Paradigm of Youth Violence Prevention. Am J Public Health 2021;111(S1):S28–31.
19. DuBose J, MacAllister L, Hadi K, et al. Exploring the Concept of Healing Spaces. Health Environments Research and Design Journal 2018;11(1):43–56.
20. Ginwright S. The Future of Healing: Shifting from Trauma Informed Care to Healing Centered Engagement. Published 2018. Medium.com. Available at: https://ginwright.medium.com/the-future-of-healing-shifting-from-traumainformed-care-to-healing-centered-engagement-634f557ce69c. Accessed March 1, 2023.
21. Barkin SL, Finch SA, Ip EH, et al. Is office-based counseling about media use, timeouts, and firearm storage effective? Results from a cluster-randomized, controlled trial. Pediatrics 2008;122(1):e15–25.
22. Purtle J, Dicker R, Cooper C, et al. Hospital-based violence intervention programs save lives and money. J Trauma Acute Care Surg 2013;75(2):331–3.
23. Rajan S, Branas CC. Arming school teachers: What do we know? Where do we go from here? Am J Public Health 2018;108(7):860–2.
24. Vossekuil B. The final report and findings of the safe school initiative: implications for the prevention of school attacks in the United States. Washington, DC: Diane Publishing; 2002.
25. Kingston B, Mattson SA, Dymnicki A, et al. Building Schools' Readiness to Implement a Comprehensive Approach to School Safety. Clin Child Fam Psychol Rev 2018;21(4):433–49.
26. David-Ferdon C, Vivolo-Kantor AM, Dahlberg LL, et al. A comprehensive technical package for the prevention of youth violence and associated risk behaviors. Published online; 2016.
27. David-Ferdon C, Simon TR. Preventing youth violence: opportunities for action. Atlanta, GA: National Center for Injury Prevention and Control, Centers for Disease Control and Prevention; 2014.
28. Gorman-Smith D, Bechhoefer D, Cosey-Gay FN, et al. A Model for Effective Community-Academic Partnerships for Youth Violence Prevention. Am J Public Health 2021;111(S1):S25–7.
29. Kingston BE, Zimmerman MA, Wendel ML, et al. Developing and Implementing Community-Level Strategies for Preventing Youth Violence in the United States. Am J Public Health 2021;111(S1):S20–4.
30. Branas CC, Kondo MC, Murphy SM, et al. Urban Blight Remediation as a Cost-Beneficial Solution to Firearm Violence. Am J Public Health 2016;e1–7.
31. D'Inverno AS, Bartholow BN. Engaging Communities in Youth Violence Prevention: Introduction and Contents. Am J Public Health 2021;111(S1):S10–6.
32. Santaella-Tenorio J, Cerdá M, Villaveces A, et al. What Do We Know About the Association Between Firearm Legislation and Firearm-Related Injuries? Epidemiol Rev 2016;38(1):140–57.
33. Fleegler EW, Lee LK, Monuteaux MC, et al. Firearm legislation and firearm-related fatalities in the United States. JAMA Intern Med 2013;173(9):732–40.
34. Lee LK, Fleegler EW, Farrell C, et al. Firearm Laws and Firearm Homicides: A Systematic Review. JAMA Intern Med 2017;177(1):106–19.
35. Siegel M, Pahn M, Xuan Z, et al. The Impact of State Firearm Laws on Homicide and Suicide Deaths in the USA, 1991–2016: a Panel Study. J Gen Intern Med 2019;34(10):2021–8.
36. Patel J, Leach-Kemon K, Curry G, et al. Firearm injury-a preventable public health issue. Lancet Public Health 2022;7(11):e976–82.

37. Rand Corporation. The Science of Gun Policy : A Critical Synthesis of Research Evidence on the Effects of Gun Policies in the United States. Available at: https://www.rand.org/pubs/research_reports/RR2088.html. Accessed March 1, 2023.

38. Díez C, Kurland RP, Rothman EF, et al. State Intimate Partner Violence–Related Firearm Laws and Intimate Partner Homicide Rates in the United States, 1991 to 2015. Ann Intern Med 2017;167(8):536–43.

39. American Academy of Pediatrics. More than 300 Pediatricians Submit Personal Testimonies of Gun Violence to Congressional Record. Available at: https://www.aap.org/en/news-room/news-releases/aap/2022/more-than-300-pediatricians-submit-personal-testimonies-of-gun-violence-to-congressional-record/#:~:text=WASHINGTON%2C%20DC%20%E2%80%93%20In%20advance%20of,their%20patients%2C%20communities%20and%20lives. Accessed March 1, 2023.

40. Everytown for Gun Safety. What is the Bipartisan Safer Communities Act? Available at: https://www.everytown.org/what-is-the-bipartisan-safer-communities-act/. Accessed March 1, 2023.

41. Cunningham RM, Ranney ML, Goldstick JE, et al. Federal funding for research on the leading causes of death among children and adolescents. Health Aff 2019; 38(10):1653–61.

42. Stark DE, Shah NH. Funding and Publication of Research on Gun Violence and Other Leading Causes of Death. JAMA 2017;317(1):84–5.

43. Bipartisan Solutions to Cyclical Violence Act. Available at: https://www.govtrack.us/congress/bills/117/s2422/text/is. Accessed March 1, 2023.

44. Dr. Guerrero's Testimony at Oversight Hearing on Gun Violence Crisis,. Available at: https://oversight.house.gov/news/press-releases/icymi-dr-guerrero-s-testimony-at-oversight-hearing-on-gun-violence-crisis. Accessed March 1, 2023.

45. Rostron A. The Dickey amendment on federal funding for research on gun violence: A Legal dissection. Am J Public Health 2018;108(7):865–7.

46. Stracqualursi V. Congress agrees to millions in gun violence research for the first time in decades. CNN.com. December 17, 2019.

47. Gun Violence Prevention Research Roundtable. Increasing FY23 Appropriations for gun violence prevention research 2022.

48. Lee LK, Douglas K, Hemenway D, et al. Crossing Lines–A Change in the Leading Cause of Death among U.S. Children. N Engl J Med 2022;386(16):1485–7.

49. Wright JL, Johnson TJ. Child Health Advocacy: The Journey to Antiracism. Pediatr Clin North Am 2023;70(1):91–101.

50. Community Catalyst. Developing and Implementing Policy Campaigns. Available at: https://www.communitycatalyst.org/resources/tools/roadmaps-to-health/developing-and-implementing-policy-campaigns. Accessed January 3, 2023.

51. Shah S. Going Farther by Going Together: Collaboration as a Tool in Advocacy. Pediatr Clin North Am 2023;70(1):181–91.

52. Pulcini CD, Raphael JL, Lopez KN. Translating Research into Child Health Policy: Aligning Incentives and Building a New Discourse. Pediatr Clin North Am 2023; 70(1):151–64.

53. Klass P, Heard-Garris N, Navsaria D. Effective Communication for Child Advocacy: Getting the Message out Beyond Clinic Walls. Pediatr Clin North Am 2023;70(1):165–79.

54. Kanak M, Turley K, Lee LK, et al. Community-Academic Advocacy to Improve Shelter Access for Families Experiencing Homelessness. Pediatrics 2023;151(2). e2022057935.

Printed and bound by CPI Group (UK) Ltd, Croydon, CR0 4YY

03/10/2024

01040471-0018